Reverse Type 2 Diabetes FOREVER!

What your doctor won't tell you about reversing Type 2 Diabetes and how you can come off your medications once and for all!

Second Edition

Dr. Laura Shwaluk B.Sc., D.C., PSc.D.

Publisher: Fun Stuff, LLC
            2540 East Plano Pkwy #142
            Plano TX 75074

ISBN 13: 978-0-9797325-3-9
ISBN 10: 0-9797325-3-0

Cover design by Jeanna Pool of "Marketing For Solos"

ACKNOWLEDGEMENTS

Thank you to all our participants who have generously shared their story to be included in this book.
Thank you Jerry, my husband, for believing in me, your understanding, and your support. You are the BEST!

CONTENTS

Introduction

Have you been diagnosed with pre-diabetes or Type 2 Diabetes? Are you sick of taking medications? Have they made you feel even worse? Are you done dragging yourself through your work days and collapsing on the couch when you get home? Do you just plain want your life back? Do you want to discover easy ways to increase your health - long term?

If you answered "Yes" to *any* of those questions, and you're willing to follow a step-by-step system for increasing your health, then this book is for you. And, like many of our participants, you might even get healthier than you *ever* remember - regardless of your genetics. On the other hand, if you are not ready or don't do the right things in the right order at the right times, you might become part of the scary high statistics about Diabetes.

According to the American Diabetes Association, 86 million Americans age 20 and older had *pre*-diabetes in 2012; this is up from 79 million in 2010. The percentage compared to the total population of the United States is 37% in 2012, and is now at 51% among those age 65 and older. That is a HUGE percentage. And part of the problem is that many never find out *how* to be healthy or believe that they *can* be healthy, resulting in diabetes still being the 7th leading cause of deaths in America.

"Yikes" is right! At least you're not alone, but this is obviously still a problem with your health.

So let's talk about healing. And let's do it like you're sitting in my office with the door closed, no time limits, and asking me whatever's on your mind. That's how this book is written: as a conversation, so you have answers to many common questions about how to be healthy, so that you can have an effect on Pre-Diabetes and Type 2 Diabetes.

But before we jump in, you might be wondering *why* I came up with a program to teach people how to increase their health, especially people with Type 2 Diabetes. I actually started as a chiropractor, helping people balance their nervous systems to make their joints, organs, glands, and life work much better. (Think of it like a full-body tune-up, which is why it's part of one of my "5 Tools of Health" I share with you in this book.) I really got interested in Type 2 Diabetes when client after client kept bringing in blood lab test results asking for help interpreting what was going on inside them. They were determined to **NOT** take medication. I got hooked on understanding it all, so I put in literally thousands of hours studying the science behind the numbers - Functional Nutrition, Functional Endocrinology, Applied Kinesiology, and more.

The more I studied, the more one thing became clear: **more people struggled with Type 2 Diabetes** (and its horrendous side effects) **than any other disease I saw**. So it became my mission to teach everyone who has it, or who is heading toward it, that there is another path to health. *You can take control of your health.*

That's still my mission. The first edition of this book was geared toward those who live near our office who could participate in our programs on location. I'm very happy to say that we heard the requests from people in other states and countries to put the 12 week "Diabetes Turning Point Program" into an online program. My commitment is to teach people all over the world, which is why the second edition of this book has more information and the online program is more accessible to everyone.

Now here's how my approach is different than a regular medical doctor. I practice what's commonly called 'functional medicine,' which is the practice of focusing on increasing health to affect the *function* of the glands and organs of your body. This addresses **underlying** root causes of health issues. I can then teach people what to do to increase their health instead of prescribing medication. In my case, I'm like the Sherlock Holmes of what's getting in the way of you being healthy. I've seen thousands of people over the years, and have found patterns in people's health that makes it easier to quickly solve mysteries other doctors couldn't figure out.

Disclaimer:

Let me be very clear, we at www.bloodsugarideas.com (NTC Health and Fitness) are functional medicine practitioners with the Pastoral Medical Association (PMA). The program's design is to educate you on maintaining your health and well-being. **The program is NOT designed to treat or cure disease, however, when the program is followed accordingly, it has been proven to enhance one's life style and health in drastic ways.**

Practitioners of Pastoral Science & Medicine offer health improvement and counseling services based on a ministerial license issued by the Pastoral Medical Association (PMA). (www.pmai.us)

PMA licensees do not practice medicine. More specifically, we do not examine, diagnose or treat, or offer to treat or cure or attempt to cure, any mental or physical disease, disorder or illness, or any physical deformity or injury. Also, PMA licensees do not recommend or prescribe any medications or pharmaceutical drugs.

Please understand that your personalized program is for the sole purpose of teaching you how to improve your functional physiology, thereby improving your everyday activities and health. Your individualized program is **NOT** intended to fully eliminate any or all dysfunctions in the time frame designed, but to proactively address your concerns so that you may become independent in the lifestyle changes that will ultimately govern your health and well being.

If you have questions regarding your prescription medications you can talk to either your doctor who prescribed the medication or your pharmacist.

You will read many stories from our participants who have had wonderful and satisfying results with their health. Not everyone will get the same results, as the results vary from person to person.

That said, functional medicine is about *you* taking personal responsibility for your health. You can't put that responsibility on me or any other doctor. You'll only get the results if you put in the work. That's why I highly suggest that your spouse, partner, boyfriend, girlfriend, or another friend read this book too and participate with you. Having a partner in the process is priceless. Your partner can help you from backsliding - especially if your partner is making lifestyle changes as you do. You'll get healthier together.

As proof, here's a couple, Dean and Nicole, in their own words about what the program did for them. Here's Dean first...

"I'm 56 years old, which means I'm on the opposite end of 50 going towards 60, so I started getting a little worried of where I was at. Before I came here, I was losing feeling in my toes. I had neuropathy. It felt like a hammer was pounding on it. I was out to here. <pointing at belly> This shirt was tight on me really.

"It must be about 5 or 6 weeks now, and I've lost about 25 pounds and gotten several inches off my belly, which is usually a hard fat because the fat's deep in there. So before I came here, I was on my deathbed. I mean, my two brothers had heart attacks that are just one year apart from me. My other brother got colon cancer. So I said, with my hereditary diabetes, my grandmother's passed away and I have several family members with diabetes, so I said,

'I'll be darned, I'm going to fight this. I can't go on diets to lose weight. I've tried that and it just didn't work.' Like Dr. Laura says, it's not just about losing weight and diet. There's a lot more to it. And so now, this is where I am. I've lost so much weight. The problem now is I'm working longer hours because I've got all this energy now!

"And I also have to say, I wouldn't be here except of course because of Dr. Laura. I'm eternally grateful. But also for my sweetheart. She's cooked foods for me that have allowed us both, as partners, to eat healthy. When you think of a diet, you think oh, bland, gross food, not enough food. I'm eating a lot of food, but I'm eating healthy food. She's been able to come up with all these new creations and concoctions, like coconut curry chicken and I'm eating these all day long, so I've got the energy, my skin feels better, and my sleep is better. Just my overall well-being is much better."

Nicole struggled with her health before the program too. Here's what she had to say…

"I had 4 spine surgeries, and with each surgery I gained 10 pounds, and I'd already put on 12 pounds prior to the first surgery. So I put on a total of 60 pounds in the 5 years that he and I have been together. Partly because we had a lot of processed foods in our house and there was a lot of depression due to the spine surgeries. I didn't have processed foods in my house prior to this, prior to me and him, and we took that out and started eating natural, whole foods. I've not only lost 26 pounds since starting this, but my pain has reduced. I felt like I had fibromyalgia, is what it's described as. Flu type symptoms and whatever. That pain has decreased so much, it's unbelievable. I'm back to my old self but even newer than my old self. So, I'm extremely grateful."

This book is based on my step-by-step 12 week "Diabetes Turning Point" online program. It consists of videos, quizzes and downloads to read with easy to follow actions to guide you on exactly how to increase your health and possibly get control of your blood sugar. Included in the program are weekly accountability phone calls to help you get the best results, ask questions and stay on track. At the end of this book I'm going to ask you to take action on your health by joining our online program.

This book is a great first step to understanding how to control your blood sugar. So, if you're ready to get healthy and stay healthy without depending on doctors or medications, let's get started. You may be pleasantly surprised how practical the process is.

Chapter 1: Diabetes Can Kill You

If you're new to having blood sugar issues (or if you're learning about it because someone you love has blood sugar issues), then let's start with some background information. Knowing what's going on will help you to start making changes toward optimal health. This chapter will cover the basic definitions of different types of blood sugar issues, what insulin is, the 3 BIG Myths about blood sugar issues, and the terrible complications of Type 2 Diabetes. You will discover the BIGGEST mistake Type 2 Diabetics make as well as pick up some actionable new tidbits even if you're already familiar with diabetes concepts and complications.

Start with the basics, Dr. Shwaluk. What exactly is blood sugar?

Blood sugar is glucose, the main sugar your body makes from the food you eat. Your bloodstream carries glucose to your cells, which they use to generate energy in your body. Excess glucose is stored in fat cells for later use. The catch is that cells can't use the glucose without insulin (more on this later).

If you're curious about the chemistry, glucose is a simple sugar (a monosaccharide). It's also known as dextrose. Your body breaks down the foods you eat in your intestines and then directly absorbs glucose into your blood, especially from simple carbohydrates like potatoes, rice, bread, cereals, and pasta. Depending on how much work it takes to break the food down, you can get a rapid increase ('spike' or 'surge') in blood glucose or a steady increase. Between meals and while you're sleeping, your body reverses the process to produce glucose from fat and protein.

Oh okay. But you mentioned cells can't even use all that blood sugar without insulin. So what's insulin and what does it do?

Keeping it simple, insulin is a hormone your pancreas makes within special 'beta cells.' Your pancreas makes insulin whenever it detects increased blood sugar (glucose), like right after eating. Every cell of your body has receptors for insulin. That means skin, liver, fat, kidney, nerve, intestines, bone, cartilage, etc. all have receptors for insulin. Glucose needs insulin as a sort of key that opens a door to let it enter your cells, where the sugar can then be used for energy - or in the case of fat cells stored for future use.

I get that diabetes is when my blood sugar is too high, and insulin plays some role in that. But what's the difference between Type 1 and Type 2 Diabetes?

Some people don't make insulin. That's called Type 1 Diabetes. It usually happens early in life, which is why it's also called 'juvenile diabetes.' Many studies are indicating that Type 1 Diabetes is actually an auto-immune disease, where a person's own immune system attacks and destroys the beta cells that make insulin.

Type 2 Diabetes, on the other hand usually happens later in life, and is when your cells stop responding normally to the insulin that your body produces. They just no longer recognize insulin very well anymore, which is why Type 2 Diabetes is also called 'Insulin Resistant' diabetes. Type 1 and Type 2 Diabetes can both cause dangerously high blood sugar levels.

Important Note: Reducing the insulin surges, over time, helps your cells to recognize insulin better long term. The best analogy is if you wear a ring on your finger for a long period of time. Eventually you won't really notice that the ring is there. It is as though you have become resistant to the feeling. However, if you take it off for a while and then put it back on you will be able to feel that it is back on your finger. Controlling the insulin surges and glucose spike is paramount to reducing your insulin resistance and increasing your chances of getting off diabetes medications.

So are both kinds of diabetes the same as hyperglycemia? And what's hypoglycemia?

Hyperglycemia is the medical term for abnormally high blood sugar, which we just talked about. It's what people with diabetes have. Hypoglycemia is the opposite: it means abnormally low blood sugar (glucose).

Ironically, treating diabetes with medication often results in hypoglycemia, since it's easy to overdo diabetes medication. Over-exercising is another common cause. Other conditions, many of them thankfully rare, can also cause low blood sugar even in people without diabetes. Hypoglycemia isn't a disease itself, like fever, it's an indicator of a health problem.

Treating hypoglycemia means quickly getting your blood sugar level back up into a normal range, either with high-sugar foods or medications. Otherwise a person might end up in the hospital in a coma from hypoglycemia. Long-term care requires identifying and correcting the underlying cause of the hypoglycemia.

What's the progression to Type 2 Diabetes? And how do I know if I have it?

The first stage in the progression toward Type 2 Diabetes is that your normal blood sugar level (when you feel fine, have no symptoms of blood sugar issues, and your blood lab results are in normal range) drops to low blood sugar (hypoglycemia). When your blood sugar drops too low, you'll often feel lightheaded and shaky. You might also be irritable or fatigued if you miss meals. But eating normally restores your blood sugar to normal at this stage. In the next stage, you start getting signs of 'insulin resistance' or 'pre-diabetes.' That's when you start feeling tired *after* meals, you struggle to lose weight, and your waist-to-hip girth balloons. You may feel hungry and crave sweets or simple carbohydrates.

At this point, your blood lab tests showing your risk for Type 2 Diabetes (Hemoglobin A1c test) may be in the pre-diabetes range. People with pre-diabetes can have symptoms of both hypoglycemia and insulin resistance. Outright Type 2 Diabetes is the next stage in the progression, which is when your blood lab tests for glucose and Hemoglobin A1c are too high and the various complications of high blood sugar start happening.

The next stage is often called 'Double Diabetes.' This is the last stage in the diabetes progression and it happens when a person with Type 2 Diabetes stops making insulin. Effectively these people are then both Type 2 and Type 1 diabetic, requiring both pills for the insulin resistance and insulin shots.

Functional Hemoglobin A1c blood test ranges:

Hypoglycemia	= below 5.0%
Normal	= 5.0 to 5.5 %
Pre-diabetes	= 5.6 to 6.4 %
Diabetes	= 6.5 % and up

NOTE: These are the optimal (functional) lab ranges, which may be different than what you see on your test sheets from the lab. More about this is in chapter three.

All that said, there's a big caution flag here. Many people have very few or such mild symptoms that they don't even realize they have blood sugar issues. They just think their symptoms are normal because they've felt like that for so long. In our program participants fill out a Health Assessment Questionnaire, which distinguishes the difference in symptoms between the types of blood sugar issues as well as the symptoms related to all the other organs and glands. We suggest this questionnaire in addition to the simple blood test that shows your risk for Type 2 Diabetes, so you know exactly where you are on the risk scale and can then learn how to correct any issues. This is very useful in helping you recognize the symptoms of a blood sugar issue, as well as many other health issues.

On my website (www.bloodsugarideas.com) you can fill out a short version of the questionnaire about your blood sugar symptoms. It is kind of like taking a quiz to find out your risk of diabetes. Knowing these symptoms gives you an idea of whether your blood sugar is normal, low, or diabetic.

What are some causes of Type 2 Diabetes?

Let me start by saying that most people believe Type 2 Diabetes is only caused by terrible diet and lack of exercise. They are certainly contributing factors, yet they are not the only cause of Type 2 diabetes. There are many factors that can and will affect your blood sugar.

Here is a list of fourteen of the most common items that can and will affect your blood sugar:

- Eating a lot of sugar
- Stress - adrenal gland exhaustion
- Infection
- Inflammation
- Dehydration
- Trauma or Surgery
- Lack of Exercise
- Eating starchy foods - the simple carbohydrates
- Food sensitivity
- Medications - steroids and antibiotics
- Lack of sleep
- Pain
- Lack of good Probiotics
- Not enough Fiber

It's important to get to the root cause of why you have a blood sugar issue if you are going to control Type 2 Diabetes properly. Many doctors are not even aware that these items can affect blood sugar and so don't address them. These are items you will learn a lot more about in our programs.

Can Type 2 Diabetes really be reversed?

Yes! Many of our program participants have done it. And you can too!

Many diabetics just like you around the world have thrown up their hands and said, "Enough!" They no longer accept choking down one drug after another, hoping only to slow the inevitable creeping up of diabetes 'crippling complications.' All it takes to have control of your health is an easy-to-follow, step-by-step approach, ideally with an accountability partner and learning the nuances in your daily habits that can make a TREMENDOUS difference in your health.

A great example of this is a guy named Kent. In January his A1C number was at 12 percent, which was very high. Following my program taught him how to increase his health and he was able to get his A1C number down to 5.6 percent by July. This book will teach you how you, too, can likely increase your health and possibly reverse your diabetes. Putting your health on a totally new and improved path.

According to statistics from the CDC, Type 2 Diabetes is caused primarily by a sedentary lifestyle and poor eating habits. Therefore it is reasonable to believe that Type 2 Diabetes can be completely controlled or reversed in most cases. By making lifestyle changes, like adding exercise and improving your diet, and getting to the root cause of why there are blood sugar issues Type 2 diabetics can drop their glucose numbers back into the normal range. Effectively reversing the complications and side effects of high blood sugar too. I've been teaching people how to reach optimal health since 1996, so I know for a fact that it works.

People who follow the steps in this program succeed, by either reversing their diabetes completely, by slashing their medication dosages, or at a minimum, making sure their complications are less severe. Results will vary from person to person.

It is so VERY important to have control of your blood sugar levels because Type 2 Diabetes can cause serious complications (like a diabetic coma) needing emergency treatment. But even if your Type 2 Diabetes isn't severe, it can still damage your eyes, kidneys, nerves, and heart long term. We'll talk a lot more about this in a moment.

So if you've been suffering diabetes' horrible health effects, and you're sick of doctors only suggesting drug after drug, then you picked up this book at the right time. You don't have to struggle any more with fatigue just to get through your day.

Here's one of our many successful participants, Jireh, in his own words…

"By the time I was age 30, I had high blood pressure. When I got to 40, my triglycerides were going up sky high. By the time I got to 50, I had started on diabetes medications. Since my wife was a pharmacist, she got me a lot of free samples, so we lived by that, but then the medication just kept going higher and higher and higher. To me, that wasn't good, and my energy level was so low I was just struggling. By 2 o'clock every day I just wanted to go home. And so I started this program about 3 weeks ago, and my energy levels have dramatically increased.

"It's very interesting, because in 3 weeks I've lost an average of 5 pounds a week. I couldn't believe it. It's not three weeks yet, but I've lost an average of 5 pounds a week. I feel lighter, I have more energy, I don't have that lull at around 2 o'clock, and I just feel physically much better. I've gotten off my Metformin, which is great. And I've gotten off my high blood pressure medicine. In fact, this morning I took my blood pressure and it was 119 over 76 without medication. Usually the bottom number is in the 90s. And

in less than three weeks, I'm sold! I was a skeptic at the beginning, because I've been trying to diet for many years, but it hasn't done anything. The medication just kept increasing and increasing. But within these 3 weeks, it's just like wow! So, I'm sold!"

Before we started talking, you mentioned there's 3 'BIG Myths' about Type 2 Diabetes. What are they?

Yes, there are 3 BIG and potentially very dangerous myths about Type 2 Diabetes …

<u>Myth #1</u> – *"Diabetes always gets worse."*

Truth is, Type 2 Diabetes always gets worse IF you don't **do** anything about it. You've got to be proactive. If you eat and drink anything you want, without exercising don't expect that you'll be okay. Even with taking medication. According to the Centers for Disease Control (CDC), diabetes is preventable and controllable.

And in my experience, much of the time is completely reversible. That means off of your medications and your A1C number is in a healthy range. All it takes is following certain steps and you can have that control.

<u>Myth #2</u> – *"Type 2 Diabetes is genetic, you just have to learn to live with it."*

Only Type 1 Diabetes (when your body stops making insulin) is considered genetic. Type 2 Diabetes (when your body stops recognizing insulin), isn't genetic. Your body still makes insulin, but your cells don't recognize it anymore. It only *seems* like Type 2 Diabetes is a genetic issue, because who do we learn our eating and lifestyle habits from? Our parents or grandparents, usually. Or sometimes it's from our culture, given how our families eat and exercise.

Have a look at your own culture. Is there a lot of bread, rice, potatoes, pasta, corn, fast food? It is no surprise then that it seems that Type 2 Diabetes is genetic.

Lifestyle changes and healthy habits can trump those genetic tendencies 100% of the time when it comes to Type 2 Diabetes. You can reverse it yourself with proper detoxification, nutrition, exercise, hormone balance and nervous system balance, which you will learn about in chapter four.

<u>Myth #3</u> – *"As long as you take your medications, you'll be just fine."*

This is the BIGGEST MYTH OF ALL and the BIGGEST MISTAKE. Diabetes has countless complications, even if you're taking medication.

> **The biggest mistake a Type 2 Diabetic can make is to believe that you will avoid the complications of this disease because you are taking medications.**

Let's go through some of these big complications…

OBESITY

Diabetes can both cause and worsen obesity. Many people who start my programs are taking three or four different kinds of blood sugar medications; they're gaining weight and having a difficult time getting it off.

There are significant health issues with obesity that can end in early death:

- Difficulty moving
- Heart disease
- High cholesterol, triglycerides, and LDLs, and low HDLs

- Cancer, including cancer in the uterus, cervix, endometrium, ovaries, breast, colon, rectum, esophagus, liver, gallbladder, pancreas, kidney and prostate
- Breathing disorders, including sleep apnea, a potentially serious sleep disorder in which breathing repeatedly stops and starts
- Gallbladder disease
- Gynecologic problems, such as infertility and irregular periods
- Erectile dysfunction and sexual health issues
- Nonalcoholic fatty liver disease, a condition in which fat builds up in the liver and can cause inflammation or scarring
- Osteoarthritis
- Skin conditions, including poor wound healing
- High blood pressure

Is Type 2 Diabetes making me fat?

Yes, Type 2 Diabetes could be making you fat. It is frustrating, yet true for the majority of Type 2 Diabetics. Here's why…

Insulin is one of the three main fat-storing hormones. Its job is to take glucose out of your bloodstream to put it into your cells, especially your fat cells. When your insulin level is high, which is most commonly the case in the beginning stages of Type 2 Diabetes your body does not get the signal to burn fat. So, yes, having Type 2 Diabetes is making you fat *and* making it harder for you to lose the weight. Frustrating, right? Especially if you've been told to lose weight to help control your diabetes. Sometimes people gain weight very quickly when they start taking diabetes medications, because glucose is forced inside the fat cells.

DOUBLE DIABETES

Not everyone with Type 2 Diabetes is obese. Some are actually underweight, a sign that glucose is NOT getting inside the cells of their body. In these cases it means they've gone so long without proper blood sugar balance that their bodies are not only unable to recognize insulin (Type 2 Diabetes), but their bodies may not be making insulin anymore (Type 1 Diabetes).

This is often called 'Double Diabetes,' which is a condition where you have to take pills for the insulin resistance AND insulin shots to make up for the fact the your body is no longer making insulin. It is like a combination of Type 2 Diabetes followed later on by Type 1 Diabetes.

The theory behind how Double Diabetes happens is that eating a lot of simple carbohydrates and sugar will spike your blood glucose, causing your insulin production to rise sharply. Your body may eventually stop being able to make insulin altogether, because of the high production demand. When your body stops making insulin it is effectively like Type 1 Diabetes. At this point, even taking insulin injections may not help, since your cells are already so insulin resistant (Type 2 Diabetes). The insulin production and effectiveness just peters out.

This is a gravely serious condition! Unlike Type 1 Diabetes, simply giving insulin shots won't work, not for long. It is more complex than simply taking insulin shots. In this scenario, tight regulation of foods, exercise, and keeping a close watch on glucose numbers, as well as specific supplements and taking actions to be healthy, can often still turn it around and make a big difference.

NEUROPATHY

Another significant issue diabetes causes is *neuropathy* - a type of nerve damage. It can feel like anything from numbness, to 'pins and needles', to a nagging sharp ache. These feelings can haunt you 24 hours a day, 7 days a week, often preventing people from sleeping. Neuropathy is often in the feet, moving painfully up the legs, and sometimes in the hands. Neuropathy is unrelenting, draining a person's energy, vitality, and patience. Even the slightest added stress can easily set off more irritability.

Diabetic neuropathy can affect your digestive system, urinary tract, blood vessels and heart. For some people, these symptoms are mild; for others, the symptoms can be painful, disabling, and even fatal. That's why it's tragic that neuropathy is so common for diabetics. Especially because neuropathy can often be prevented, reversed completely or at least the progress can be slowed with tight blood sugar control and a healthy lifestyle.

PERIPHERAL ARTERY DISEASE (PAD)

Another common complication of diabetes is ***peripheral vascular disease*** (also called peripheral arterial disease), a circulatory problem in which narrowed arteries reduce blood flow to your limbs. When you develop peripheral artery disease (PAD), your extremities (usually your legs) don't get enough blood flow to keep up with demand. So you get symptoms like leg pain when you're walking. The blood flow gets so restricted that the tissues die, gangrene sets in and your foot, leg, or hand must be amputated.

Peripheral artery disease is also likely to point to more widespread fatty deposits in your arteries (atherosclerosis). You may have less blood flow to your heart, kidneys, brain, and your legs. The results can be gruesome. To give you 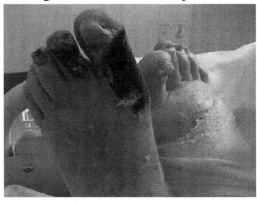 an idea, take a look at this picture from: http://www.northernsydneyvascular.com.au/PeripheralVascularDis ease.html showing a normal foot versus one with PAD.

Amputation is NOT reversible. However you can successfully prevent peripheral artery disease by reversing Type 2 Diabetes. **If you're a smoker, you'll need to quit tobacco.** Don't wait until it's too late. Many people who do our programs have a family member who had amputations because of Type 2 Diabetes. Their grandfather, grandmother, uncle, aunt, or parent had to have fingers, toes, both legs, or an arm removed. So now they can't walk or take care of themselves.

People tell me how they saw their loved one suffering, constantly dependent on others to help them with basic daily living. They can no longer work to support themselves or have the quality of life or freedom to do and go where they want, both physically and financially.

When I first started working with one particular 14-year-old-girl with Type 2 Diabetes, I asked her, "Why are you here?" If you've been around teenagers, you probably know how much they resist change unless they feel like the change is their idea. So, I asked her mom not to say anything because I wanted to know from the teen why she wanted to be in our program. And she said, "My grandmother lost both of her legs to Type 2 Diabetes, and I don't want to be in a wheelchair like she is." WOW, like I said, tragic.

KIDNEY FAILURE

Kidney destruction is one of the deadly side effects of diabetes. It is the number one complication that can kill you. Since your kidneys filter out excess fluid and toxic waste from your blood, losing this critical ability means dangerous levels of fluid and toxic waste build up in your body. That's kidney failure. People often have to go for dialysis every two to three days to have their blood filtered by a machine. But even then the dialysis machines aren't doing your kidneys' full job, so people eventually die of kidney failure anyway.

HEART ATTACK AND STROKE

Heart attack and stroke are next on the cringe-worthy list of complications. Even worse, the Centers for Disease Control and Prevention (CDC) says Type 2 Diabetes is the *top* risk factor for this **leading cause of death** for both men and women. Many of the heart attacks and strokes from Type 2 Diabetes happen because the blood vessels become so narrow, as described in the Peripheral Arterial Disease section above, and the blood becomes thick and viscous. These two issues block blood from getting to your heart and brain, therefore causing a heart attack or stroke.

Reducing blood sugar issues means you can help prevent yourself from having a heart attack or stroke. There could be other factors, such as cholesterol and inflammation in your blood stream to address as well, yet these you also have some control over. So, heart attacks and strokes are largely preventable!

This is so important, because if you've got a history of heart attacks or strokes in your family you can make a big difference in going down a different, much healthier path.

BLINDNESS

The CDC lists diabetic retinopathy (DR) as ***the leading cause of blindness in American adults age 20-74***. Diabetic retinopathy is when there is damage to the blood vessels of the light-sensitive tissue at the back of the eye (retina) - usually in both eyes. It's scary how this is an all too common diabetic side effect, and it can happen overnight. An example of what vision looks like with diabetic retinopathy is seen here in the comparison of normal vision to the black blotches blocking vision. (Taken from http://www.vincett.com/diabetic-retinopathy.html)

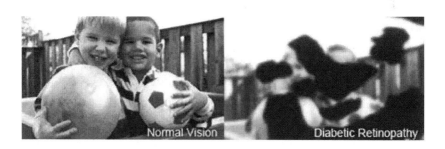

You can reduce your diabetic retinopathy risk by diagnosing it early, then controlling your blood sugar, blood pressure, and lipid abnormalities (cholesterol, triglycerides, LDH and HDL). Unfortunately, up to 50% of people don't get their eyes checked, or they're diagnosed too late for programs to be effective. Get your eyes checked once a year and protect your vision by keeping your blood sugar under control.

What is the risk if I'm not proactive?

I hope that you are now inspired to make the simple changes needed to avoid those Type 2 Diabetes horrors. You now know that taking medication alone isn't remotely near enough to prevent the complications. You risk becoming disabled and a physical burden to your family. If you do have a stroke, go blind, or lose your legs, who will take care of you? How will you support yourself and your family if you aren't able to carry on? I urge you to be proactive *before* you cause a physical and financial calamity to yourself and your family.

Chapter 2: Done Feeling Tired?

This chapter covers many common questions people have about reversing Type 2 Diabetes. You'll learn about your fatigue, weight, thirst, sleep, sugar cravings, and how long it really takes (on average) to turn Type 2 Diabetes around. For a complete list of symptoms of abnormal blood sugar levels, you can fill out the quiz at www.bloodsugarideas.com

Will I ever get my energy back? I'm so tired all the time, and I need to do more than ever just to take care of myself.

I hear you. Fatigue is the number one reason people seek help. They feel like they can barely get through the day. When they get home from work, they're so tired they can't do anything or don't want to do anything. Sometimes they go straight to sleep on the sofa for an hour or two, and then get up to have their evening meal. Even then, they only have enough energy to watch TV or do something mindless that hardly takes any energy. They stop being with friends and family or doing the things they used to love doing. They're just *existing*, not *living*.

When I ask our program participants who have Type 2 Diabetes how much energy they have on average every day (with 0% = no energy and 100% = full energy) they often say about 50 to 60%, sometimes less. It's that deep tiredness that stops people from living a quality life, filled with love, adventure, and being of service.

Carol, a program participant, said...

"I'm frightened that I'm going to die the way my mother did, so I feel that I have to do something about it now. I feel numb to life and doing things in life, and if that is what living is then I don't want to live anymore.

I want to be able to do my hobbies, volunteer, travel and spend time with my family, yet I just don't seem to have the energy, and that makes me feel down ever further."

To keep your commitment to increasing your health, always remember your reasons for wanting to be healthy: being able to spend time with your children or grandchildren, avoiding serious health complications, avoiding becoming a burden to your family, getting off your medications.

You aren't too tired to start. I promise. Even though it may feel like it right now. And you'll find it easier and easier to follow the program when you start seeing and feeling the results (often in the very first weeks).

No doubt fatigue makes you miss being able to do things you love with the people you love. And you want to do those things with the mental clarity to think and laugh and really make a difference in your life and the world. Most people start feeling their best anywhere between 3 and 10 weeks after starting the program, routinely telling me things like "I feel more energetic than I've ever felt in my life."

Here's what Victor, age 56, had to say about his experience in my 12 week program...

"I've had Type 2 Diabetes for about 8 years now and when I first started, my glucose readings were close to 500. In those 8 years I started with Metformin, 500 mgs, and then 1000 mgs, and then twice a day. Then my doctor put me on Actos and said it was a great thing for me, it will help me, it will lower my levels. Then I started on Januvia, and I was still taking Actos and Metformin. Then I went to insulin shots and last year I went to Lantus, and that wasn't working and so she said what I need was Humalog. I felt like I was just chasing myself with all these drugs.

I was feeling tired. I was so stressed. I thought it was work that was stressing me out, and of course that's part of it, but I think that my internal feeling and chemistry was just so bad that I couldn't control stress. It was just shooting my levels up, more insulin, more Humalog, and I was just constantly feeling really bad. I didn't feel like doing anything. I just wanted to get home, sleep, and worry about trying to get up in the morning and going to work.

About 6 months ago, I went to the doctor and my A1c was 8.9 percent. Then three months ago, I went into this 'I'm gonna do it myself.' I'm gonna eat veggies and fruit and I'm gonna do it on my own cause I'm tired of this medication 'phase', and I think this last visit was 7.9 - 8.1, which was better, but not enough.

This Tuesday was three weeks ago that I started my program to reverse Type 2 Diabetes with Dr. Shwaluk. My wife dragged me along. She doesn't have diabetes, but she was always trying to control weight and feel good, but she was tired all the time too. So I finally said, you know what? If you want to do it, I'll do it with you. Because for the past 8 years, I would lose weight a little bit but my sugar level was still bad. So this time we decided that we would do it together.

I came in with some reservations. The first couple days are the testing part, where we're figuring out the root cause of the problem. She does a good analysis of that. Then I started my detoxification three weeks ago and I was still taking those 5 medications. I was probably paying $300 a month just for *medications.*

The first week of the detox I was just trying to get adjusted to the changes. It was surprising. I was seeing my waking up fasting glucose readings go from 180 down to 89-90. That's another good thing, you don't have to be checking your levels constantly anymore. Dr. Shwaluk told me to consult with my doctor on how I should get off my medication, if I saw that my numbers were going down.

Now my fasting blood sugar is at about 73 to 83 and I'm down to one medication. In fact, the last two days I didn't need it anymore either and I'm still averaging in that 80 range. The program that she has me on, it's amazing. In the last three weeks, I've become energetic and I can move easily. I've got 4- and 5- year old grandkids who like to run, and before, my joints were to a point where I would move my hands and they would lock up. I don't have any more locking sensation. I was getting scared, 'cause like Dr. Shwaluk said in the presentation, 'who do you live for?' And I was like, man now I'm not gonna get to see them as they grow.

The weight loss isn't really what I was here for, but I've lost 14 pounds in these three weeks. So the weight loss is a secondary thing to me, but the main thing is how awesome it is to feel good. The insulin and drugs and all that being gone is fantastic, but the biggest thing to me is that I don't crash in my energy anymore. I used to run around every day to get a candy bar so I wouldn't get shaky and nervous. Now I can wait for lunch until almost 2 and then my body says, 'Hey, you're hungry'. But I'm not crashing. I'm eating, but not living to eat. I have time to enjoy myself. I'm happy! I'm smiling! Thank you so much for what you've done for us. Thank you so much."

That really gives me some hope, Dr. Shwaluk. Tell me *why* I feel so tired? I want to understand.

The main reason you may be feeling tired is because your cells don't recognize the insulin anymore that your pancreas is creating.

Any and all cells are affected by insulin resistance, liver, muscle, brain, nerve, bone, kidney, skin, etc. So the glucose in your blood can't get into the cells to generate energy. No glucose equals no energy. Simple as that. It's also why, ironically, you may feel even more tired *after* meals. Your body creates extra insulin to shuttle the sugar into your cells, but it can't get it into the cells, which causes an extra load on your system.

There are other reasons for fatigue related to Type 2 Diabetes, like not sleeping well from the pain of neuropathy or having to wake up in the night multiple times to pee. Additional issues related to Type 2 Diabetes fatigue also include: dehydration, adrenal exhaustion, food sensitivities, the medications you are taking, or your body trying to heal from the damaging side effects of Type 2 Diabetes. All of these can drag your energy down.

Different people also get tired at different times of the day. Many people feel sleepy in the middle of the afternoon. Some people have a hard time getting up in the morning. Whatever your energy cycle, with Type 2 Diabetes you might feel like you've hardly got the energy to get through your day.

Makes sense. But will I become even more tired when I start your program? I can't afford to be a total zombie.

Most people start to feel more energetic in the first weeks of the program. However, sometimes people do feel more tired when they start any program to increase their health.

Although rare, here are three reasons why someone might feel tired the first one to two weeks of their program:

1.   One is that your body isn't used to making a fat-burning hormone called glucagon anymore - the main fat burning hormone. When your blood sugar first goes back to normal, your body needs retraining time to start burning fat instead of only burning simple sugars. That's why you may feel like you need a sugar fix. Watch out for thoughts like, "If I could just have a donut or candy bar or a Coke or something, I'll get my

energy back." Don't cave into those cravings. Give it some time. Your reward will be predictably consistent energy all day long.

2.　　　The second reason for fatigue when someone first starts any program is because healing tissues, plus repairing organs and glands, requires the extra energy. Remember from chapter one that Type 2 Diabetes is extremely destructive to your body, including nerves, arteries, skin, brain, kidneys, heart, etc. As soon as your body has the opportunity to heal, it'll take it even though it might make you feel tired. Again, your reward for slowing down a little will be speeding up soon and for the long term.

3.　　　The third reason is similar to the second, because a good program starts with detoxification. Any kind of detox takes energy to rid your body of all the dangerous toxic buildup - environmental pollution, preservatives, previous medications, etc. That said, most people don't notice this one as much as the first two. You'll learn more about detoxification in chapter four.

That sounds like a short-term price worth paying. But why am I thirsty all the time right now?

Given all the excess sugar in your blood, your kidneys are forced to work overtime to filter and remove the excess sugar. That sugar is excreted into your urine along with fluids drawn from your tissues. This triggers more frequent urination, which may leave you dehydrated and feeling thirsty.

Ahh, so I'll actually be less thirsty on your program. Will I shed some weight too?

Most people lose 10 to 20 pounds in the first four weeks on the program and then weight loss happens a little more slowly after that. You will probably lose weight if you need to, because a healthy body isn't an overweight body. Many people have it backwards when it comes to losing weight. They believe they'd be healthy if they could just lose weight first. However, getting healthy using good nutrition, good nutraceuticals (vitamin/ mineral/ herbal formulations), detoxification, hormone balance, and plenty of exercise, gets you healthy and lets the weight naturally come off.

That is, if you even have extra weight to lose. If you don't have extra weight to lose, then you just need to get healthy and perhaps gain some muscle mass back. Either way, the more normal your weight is, the easier it is to manage your blood sugar levels. That's part of how you can come down off your medications. It's exciting to watch people become healthy again - and then become healthier than they can ever remember. They don't have any more weight "yo-yo" ups and downs because they know how to stay healthy once the program is over.

Will I start sleeping better too?

Sleeping better is one of the most common and appreciated benefits to controlling your blood sugar and increasing your health. Are you one of those people who often wakes up in the night and can't fall back asleep for half an hour or more? Or you need to get up multiple times to pee? Your blood sugar is probably off if this happens to you. Deeper and longer sleep feels like a luxury if you've been without it for a while, and many people sleep much better within weeks of starting the 12 week program.

"Just want to say thanks and let you know how great I'm doing. Before starting your program I was just feeling "blah" all the time. Never wanted to do ANYTHING!

Now it seems I am happier and sleeping sooooooo much better! Also I am losing weight! The best part is that I WILL NOT need to be put on medicine and I will be here to enjoy my life and family!!!"

Patricia P. Age 65 Plano, TX

Better sleep, weight loss, and less nagging thirst… You've got my attention now. Will I also stop having sugar cravings?

Sugar cravings and hunger are very common with Type 2 Diabetes. A few of our participants, like Lisa, have told me things like *"I know where every donut shop is in the city"* because they have such terrible cravings. If you're purposely running errands near donut shops (or other places selling sugary junk), you know what I mean. Because your cells don't recognize insulin they aren't getting enough glucose, resulting in you feeling hungry. The cells send powerful signals to your brain compelling you to eat simple sugars including simple carbohydrates such as bread, rice, pasta, cereals, or potatoes. Of course, that only makes the situation worse. Your body makes even more insulin to clear out the dangerous amount of glucose, but that insulin isn't recognized either. It's a vicious cycle.

On my program, the sugar cravings usually stop within the first 2 weeks. If they don't, you may have an infection like yeast, fungi, or bacteria, which can also send powerful signals to your brain to eat sugar or simple carbohydrates. This is what was happening with Lisa. She would wake up in the morning thinking about what type of sugar she was going to eat for breakfast, lunch and dinner. Planned her whole day around where she was going to buy it and how she was going to hide it from her husband. The sugar cravings quickly went away when the infection was knocked out. She said it was like a 'miracle' that she no longer craved sugar.

On average, how long does it take to reverse Type 2 Diabetes?

There isn't a definitive answer, because it depends on your current health, how old you are, if you're taking medications (including how long you've been taking those medications and how many you're taking), your current eating and exercise habits, how healthy your tissues are, how coachable you are, and how committed you are to achieving your health goals. Some of our participants have turned their health around in only three or four months, like Jireh who you've already read about. Others have taken 12 months or more, like Dale who is steadily working at improving his health day by day. Chipping away at it a bit at a time.

It takes constant work to stay on right track but is do able and I feel a lot better and do not have to rely on drugs that were not working anyway. It requires a change of life-long habits that is the hardest part, but the results are worth the hard work.

Mark E. Plano, TX

Chapter 3: What Doctors Can't Tell You

In this chapter you'll learn the link between cholesterol and diabetes, how the healthcare industry has you trapped, what Hemoglobin A1C really means, and what's required to get on the road to optimal health.

"I started this program in mid April 2014. I was taking 2 pills plus 2 insulin shots a day for diabetes, plus medicine for cholesterol, high blood pressure, acid reflux, and high triglycerides when I started.

Now 3 1/2 months later, I have lost 28 pounds, cut out 1 diabetic pill plus 1 insulin, reduced other insulin by half, cut out meds for acid reflux, triglycerides and reduced a couple of other meds.

I feel great! Although I still sometimes run out of energy before the end of the day, I am able to do a lot more physical activities than I have done in a long time. (including some exercise)

With determination and lots of encouragement this has been relatively easy to follow. We have traveled a lot and moved out of

*state since starting the program and although it's been a
challenge at times, I've been able to stick with it.*

*I still have several months to go before I reach my goal of getting
rid of my diabetes medicines and losing another 15 pounds, but I
know with this program and Dr. Laura's knowledge and support, I
will make it!"*

Carol W.   Age 65   Mountain Home, AR

How come no one told me about this before?

What participants are referring to when they ask that question is,
*"Why didn't my medical doctor tell me how to prevent Type 2
Diabetes? Or teach me how reverse it?"*

Most medical doctors want you to be healthy, but they're mostly
trained to prescribe medication. They often don't *want* to give you
more pills, but it's what they've been taught. They haven't been
trained on how to help you naturally balance your blood sugar
once it's out of whack, and they don't get paid by insurance to
educate people about optimal health. Yes, there are exceptions,
just like with everything, but you probably wouldn't be reading
this if your doctor was one of the exceptions. In their defense,
medical doctors *do* often say *"watch your diet and get some
exercise."* They just don't have the specifics of which foods to eat,
how often to eat, which kinds of exercise or detoxification would
be best, or how to balance hormones in natural ways that don't
require prescription medication.

The *British Medical Journal* stated that "Eighty-five percent of all
medical procedures and surgeries are scientifically unproven."
That's a bold statement. What they were referring to is chronic
disease, including conditions like Type 2 Diabetes,
hypothyroidism, gastrointestinal problems, heart disease, cancer,
obesity, and auto-immune diseases. A **chronic disease** is one
lasting 3 months or more, by the definition of the U.S. National

Center for Health Statistics. Chronic diseases generally can't be prevented by vaccines or cured by medications, nor do they just disappear. These are among the most slow-growing, costly, devastating and yet *preventable* of all health problems.

The other fifteen percent of medical procedures and surgeries, where medical doctors *are* highly efficient and effective, is in 'acute conditions.'

These are sudden issues you might go to the emergency room for, such as a broken leg, severe burn, deep cut, or car crash. Other acute issues include heart attack, stroke, appendicitis or heat stroke

One of my brothers is an emergency room doctor, so I know how amazing medical doctors are when treating what they're good at. Please don't think I'm against medical doctors. What I'm *for* is people taking charge of their health.

So if I can't blame my doctor, who can I blame for not making the proper info available?

Health insurance companies are part of the problem. There's an excellent movie called *"Escape Fire – The Fight to Rescue American Healthcare"* that puts the healthcare system and health insurance into perspective. If you watch the trailer at http://www.escapefiremovie.com, you'll get a sense of how the medical doctors are trapped in a system that's broken, and it's only going to make us worse. Because the doctors are trapped, who else is trapped too? All of us.

Insurance won't pay for proactive or true preventative care, so doctors and hospitals don't provide the service. What *does* insurance pay for? Insurance pays for some doctor visits and emergency services. It also pays for some lab and diagnostic tests for the acute conditions mentioned above. Does it help you pay for good, healthy organic foods? Does it pay your gym membership? How about an education - a program for you to learn how to be healthy? Insurance doesn't cover these things. Insurance was not made for these things, it was developed for acute care. Relying on what insurance covers when is come to chronic disease is a big part of why people are getting sicker and sicker.

At the time of publishing this book, if you live in the United States of America, you are required to have health insurance or pay a penalty. Are you automatically going to become healthier as a result of having insurance? No, of course not. The bottom line is that it's up to you to take your health into your own hands. Nothing will change unless you take action to make a change.

Well said. That's a great perspective to have. Getting into diabetes' offshoot effects, is cholesterol linked to diabetes?

Yes, your blood sugar level impacts your cholesterol. Here's the gist of how it works... Insulin doesn't just regulate your blood sugar. Did you know it also regulates fats? But because fat, liver and muscle cells don't recognize insulin when you've got Type 2 Diabetes, the insulin builds up in your blood.

High insulin blocks your body from burning fat for energy by blocking glucagon release. Glucagon is a hormone your pancreas creates to help break down fat to glucose in the liver. In other words, glucagon helps you break down fat to glucose when your blood sugar levels get low - this helps you lose weight. When there's too much insulin, your pancreas doesn't make enough glucagon. Therefore, fatty compounds like cholesterol, triglycerides, and LDL's build up in your liver. In fact, high cholesterol and triglycerides are one of the first red flags for Type 2 Diabetes in your blood work. They often signal that you're developing diabetes. If fats keep building up in your liver, you get the condition called 'Fatty Liver.' Left unchecked, you'll eventually have 'Metabolic Syndrome.'

Metabolic Syndrome is actually a cluster of conditions - increased blood pressure, high blood sugar, excess body fat around your waist, and abnormal cholesterol levels - that occur together, increasing your risk of heart disease, stroke, and diabetes. Having just one of these conditions doesn't mean you have Metabolic Syndrome. However, any of these conditions increase your risk of serious disease. If more than one of these conditions occur in combination, your risk is even greater. If you have Metabolic Syndrome or any of its components, aggressive lifestyle changes can delay or even prevent serious health problems.

This is really good news because you can prevent or reverse Type 2 Diabetes while also getting your cholesterol and blood pressure in line. Mike is a perfect example. He was overweight, taking cholesterol and blood pressure medications for almost 25 years and was in the pre-diabetic range. He complained of stiff joints and very limited energy. It took eight months, yet he is now off both of the medications and his Hemoglobin A1C and glucose are in normal range. He lost 45 lbs, has no joint pain, increased energy level, feels better and has more self confidence with his physical appearance. This is a good example of how he took what he learned and gained health for life to have freedom from taking drugs.

Drug-free is how I want to be, so that sounds good to me! Tell me more about my Hemoglobin A1C?

The Hemoglobin A1C test is a common blood test used to diagnose both Type 1 and Type 2 Diabetes, and then to gauge how well you're managing your blood sugar. (Note that this test goes by many other names, including 'glycated hemoglobin,' 'glycosylated hemoglobin,' 'hemoglobin A1C' and 'HbA1c')

The Hemoglobin A1C test gives you an idea of your average blood sugar level for the past two to three months. It does that by measuring what percentage of your hemoglobin - the oxygen-carrying protein in your red blood cells - is coated with sugar ('glycated'). The higher your A1C level is, the worse your blood sugar control and the higher your risk of diabetes complications.

So why did my doctor tell me my A1C was normal when I have all these symptoms of blood sugar issues?

It's because what's considered normal is a wide range. Most labs consider A1C between 4.0 to 5.6 percent 'normal.' They label the range from 5.7 to 6.4 percent 'pre-diabetes,' and they call 6.5 percent and up 'diabetic.'

As a functional medicine I doctor look at the *functional* **ranges** of lab tests instead of the regular lab ranges. Let me explain. The functional lab ranges are the ranges of lab tests of healthy people who do NOT have any disease symptoms. The functional lab range for A1C is 5.0 to 5.5 percent.

Another example is the 'regular' blood lab range for glucose, in which below 70 mg/dl is considered abnormally low and above 99 mg/dl is called abnormally high. Well, the functional lab range is 85 to 99 mg/dl where people have normal blood sugar levels and NO symptoms of blood sugar issues. Straying outside of that range may not indicate you need medication, but you'll certainly have symptoms to signal that you need to do something to increase your health so that you don't end up taking medication.

Many people have been told they're 'pre-diabetic,' in that 5.6 to 6.5 percent A1C range, so they're told to watch their diets and do some exercise. But how do most people react to that advice? They do something for a while and then go back to their normal habits, or they ignore it entirely because they simply don't know how to make changes or realize the complications of Type 2 Diabetes. Worse than that, they're often told, *"You're in the pre-diabetic range, so we're going to monitor this for three to six months and then test it again."*

Now imagine you're in your front yard with your children, grandchildren, or you're watching over your friend's grandchildren. Let's say the children are about 4 or 5 years old. Imagine they see their friends in the yard across the street from your house and they say, *"Hey there's our friends!"* And then they start running toward the street to cross the street to play with their friends AND you see a car coming. What would you do? You would go after them! You're going to scream, *"Stop!"* or grab hold of them. You're not going to sit back and say, *"Well, let's just wait and see what happens. They're not at the street yet."* They are 'pre-street,' like as in 'pre-diabetes.' No, NOW is the time to reverse diabetes symptoms. Before any damage occurs.

So, if you've been told that you're pre-diabetic or recently diabetic, this is the best time to reverse it. This is the time when it's the easiest and have the longest lasting effect. Don't wait until your A1C pops over 6.5 percent and then resort to medication. By that time you're already developing the damaging blood sugar complications discussed in chapter one.

Knowing where your lab numbers line up with the functional lab numbers is extremely important. This is where you look for anything *"headed for the street."* Look at all the blood lab work to compare your numbers to the optimal functional lab ranges. Since optimal lab ranges are narrower than the typical ranges used, you will be able to spot red flags pretty quickly. The best way to learn about your health is to actually learn how to do things for yourself. That's why a section in my program is called 'Know Your Labs,' where you learn the functional ranges of the most common items tested in blood lab tests and what to do about them if they are out of range.

Reminds me of a Chinese proverb… *"Tell me and I may remember. Show me and I will remember. Involve me and I will understand."*

That's a great proverb. Let's break it down into its components. *"Tell me and I may remember..."* Do you know the percentage of information you will remember 2 days from now about what you learned in this book?

It's actually only about 7%. Forty Eight hours from now most people will only remember about 7% of what they just learned. Now, *"...show me and I will remember..."* Let's just say that you are reading a book on how to ride a bicycle. I know that's a really simple analogy but if you were reading this book and then went to my website to watch a video on how to ride a bicycle, you'd probably remember what that looked like. BUT you wouldn't feel what it's like to have balance on a bicycle until you actively do it yourself. You have to actually get on the bicycle and experience it for yourself – what that balance with your *health* feels like.

Your *involvement* is how you understand, and that's what it takes for you to be successful with your health.

Can I really predict the future of my health?

When it comes to increasing your health and controlling Type 2 Diabetes, you absolutely can - if you're following a proven system, step by step. Step one is to order the correct lab tests. Nearly 100% of the time, there are critical test results missing when people have lab work done through another doctor. Iron, C-reactive protein, vitamin D, or even A1C are commonly missing tests. Many doctors don't realize that a food sensitivity can cause Type 2 Diabetes, so don't even know to test for the issue. Bottom line is we start with getting the correct lab tests completed.

The second step is to find the underlying cause of the health issue. You can correct the issue if you focus on the cause instead of the symptoms. It is important to get to the root cause of why you have a health issue so you can fix it, rather than just altering the lab results with medication.

The third step is to address your body as a whole, using a systemized approach which you'll learn more about in the next chapter.

And the final step is having a mentor to teach you and hold you accountable, like one of our Accountability Partners that help you follow my program.

I'm your mentor, your teacher, so here is another analogy, and I'm going to give my husband credit for this one because he is the one who came up with it.

He explained that it's like you're driving in your car and the engine light comes on. Does it ever happen at a convenient time? No, just like health issues don't happen at a convenient time. Ugh! Okay. So we take the car over to the auto repair shop and say "*my engine light is on"* and they say, *"Oh, that light is bothering you? No problem, we'll just cover it up with a piece of cardboard. That light will not bother you anymore."*

Would you put up with that at the auto repair place with your car? No, we wouldn't stand for that with our car yet we do that with our body when we take pills.

Or here's another one, *"Oh the light is bothering you? Well, we'll just take that light bulb right out. That light will never bother you ever again."*

No, we wouldn't stand for that either. We need to change the oil, change the filter, or get to the root cause of why the engine light came on. It's like getting to the root cause of health issues to get your body running like the well oiled machine it was meant to be. As well as help you to lose weight, get your energy back, get off medications, and help you to feel like your normal self again. To teach you what to do, so that you really can fulfill your purpose in life.

"I was taking eight diabetic pills a day. Now I am taking one pill a day. I'm so happy, I can hardly believe I'm getting rid of those pills!"

George M.   Age 80   Allen, TX

Chapter 4: Turn It Around SYSTEM

How do I get started increasing my health?

In the previous chapter, we talked about increasing your health using a proven step-by-step system. Starting with ordering the correct lab tests (step one), then finding the underlying cause (step two), then addressing the body as a whole (step three), using a systemized approach (step four), which you will learn more about in this chapter.

"My glucose reading this morning was at 112. I'm so excited. I've never had a reading that low before. We are getting there. Just thought I would share! Have a great weekend!!"

Cynthia S. Age58 Fort Worth, TX

Many people have tried countless nutrition programs and failed. Each program might've worked for a little while, but then they end up back where they started. This is what happens with many nutrition programs. People also take nutrition classes specifically for Type 2 Diabetes, but what happens after that? Maybe they were told to exercise, but they weren't taught how to exercise properly. There wasn't any specific system to follow.

According to Dr. W. Edwards Deming, the statistics scholar and prolific writer, 94% of all failure is due to not having a system. This applies to everything in life, from business and marketing to running a household. There must be a system to succeed.

This chapter is dedicated to listing and explaining what we call the "5 Tools of Health." These are the five main areas to focus on to create optimal health. Briefly, they are Detoxification, Diet, Exercise, Hormone Balance, and the Nervous System Balance.

Tool of Health #1 - Detoxification

Why is 'detoxifying' my body so important before changing my eating and lifestyle habits?

First, you've got to detoxify your liver because all hormones and nutrients go through your liver in some way, shape, or form. So if your liver is full of toxins, or if it's sluggish for any reason, there's no way you can get all the changes in health that you want. There's no way that changing your diet, taking a specific herbal vitamin, mineral, or supplement for your blood sugar issues will work effectively. Your body won't be able to absorb or use those supplements properly.

Next, you've got to detoxify your intestines, also called your digestive tract. If you have heartburn, gas, bloating, constipation, or diarrhea, you probably aren't digesting food properly. You may have an infection or many infections. You may also have food sensitivities. One of the most common reasons people have Type 2 Diabetes is a food sensitivity causing what's called *'leaky gut.'* Having a leaky gut, in turn, causes a cascading series of events starting with inflammation, and later adrenal exhaustion, all causing your cells to stop recognizing insulin.

Many people are worried about detoxifying because they've either tried a detox program before, or they've heard other people's experiences, which sounded uncomfortable or downright scary.

But the detoxification I'm talking about is not a fast or purge, it is simply giving your body the nutrients it needs to detoxify on its own. You won't have to chain yourself to the toilet, afraid to leave the house. We suggest simple detoxification powders you mix with water and drink. Many supplement brands have a detoxification powder. You can ask one of your local natural licensed health providers for help in picking out the right one for you. Please do not just ask the clerk in a health food store who is not trained and licensed to provide suggestions.

Detoxification also includes removing toxic foods from your diet. Including anything that would cause your blood sugar to go up, such as refined sugars and simple starchy foods. They may have caused your downward spiral into Type 2 Diabetes to begin with.

You'll also stop eating the foods that people are most commonly sensitive to. Gluten is a good example. Gluten is a protein found in wheat and many other grains. People who are sensitive to gluten have symptoms similar to people with Celiac Disease - just not as severe. With a sensitivity they have antibodies against gluten and may have similar intestinal damage. Symptoms include bloating, abdominal discomfort or pain, diarrhea, constipation, muscular disturbances, headaches, migraines, severe acne, fatigue, and bone or joint pain.

*"My main objective with Dr. Laura's program was to lose weight and find out the cause of my gastrointestinal problems (severe gas, diarrhea, etc.). I've been on the program about a month now and, through the detoxification, I've been able to identify the foods that were causing my gastrointestinal problems and eliminate them from my diet. I've also started losing weight (6 pounds) and am hopeful that if I continue eating the **right** healthy foods for **me**, that I'll continue to lose the weight."*

Julie P.   Age 57   Allen, TX

One of the powders I recommend for the digestive tract is L-Glutamine. There are specific formulations to help your intestines heal from the damage food sensitivities cause and is also extremely helpful in getting rid of acid reflux.

If you are having digestive issues such as lower abdominal pain, diarrhea or constipation, bloating, stomach pain, incomplete digestion of foods, coated tongue or fuzzy debris on tongue or heartburn, then I recommend that you have a stool sample tested to find out if there is an infection. Remember, that infection and not having the right kinds of bacteria in your digestive system can cause your blood sugar numbers to rise. The appendix at the back of this book lists the GI Stool sample test as well as a number of other tests commonly recommended.

If your lab work tells you there is an infection in your digestive tract, you may need to take herbs or, in the worst cases, antibiotics to clear the infection. The next step is to reintroduce good bacteria ('probiotics') and replenish any enzymes that might've been depleted to make sure your body is healthy enough for the next step.

Probiotics and enzymes are both essential for breaking food down into particles tiny enough for your body to absorb the life-giving nutrients. What you eat and drink is your sustenance, so a healthy liver and digestive tract are critical to absorb and utilize the nutrients you eat.

"For years I sat back, like having an out of body experience, watching my life spiral into the same unhealthy path as I had seen my mother, father and many of my family of that generation as well as my own health decline. My doctors kept telling me that the cure for all my problems was in 'diet and exercise'; however what they couldn't understand was that no matter how hard I had tried and how much information I had obtained about these two topics, I still seemed to continue down the path of destruction in my health. When it seemed as though just the smell of food could put pounds on, blood pressure was beginning to become unmanageable, I was

pre-diabetic, sick for a week (which was unusual for me), tired all the time, and often experiencing digestive problems, that I begin to pray for a solution.

About two weeks later I received Dr. Laura's flyer in the mail about reversing diabetes, and I knew this was an answer to one of my problems; however little did I know that it was actually the answer to my prayers until I went to her orientation. The information that she provided was similar to some of the information I had researched on my own so I knew already that it was true. I had finally found someone that would be able to coach me back to the health that I so desired!

After 10 weeks on the program, I have lost 27 pounds (39 in total since I had started 6 weeks before starting the program looking at my food; which means that I had already lost those first easy 10 pounds and had already eliminated one food that contributed to my digestive issues unknowingly). With the elimination of several food allergies/sensitivities my digestive issues are recovering, which I understand may take several years after decades of abuse, and although I have several more weeks before I get my test results for my pre-diabetes, I know that this is also better because I no longer experience the drop in energy level throughout the day and now have enough energy to get that exercise in as well.

The 'diet and exercise' was the cure to my problems, but I needed the correct guidance and the coaching to get me through it. And guess what? With no cravings!!!! Thanks to Dr. Laura and her staff for all they do!

Luevenia R. Age 53 Allen, TX

Tool of Health #2 - Diet

I'm following the standard diabetes diet and I'm getting worse! What am I supposed to do?

There are so many myths out there about diet, especially relating to Type 2 Diabetes. Dieticians, for example, sometimes give out outdated information about Type 2 Diabetes diets. I often disagree with what they say for a couple of reasons. First, the standard diabetes diet doesn't account for the oxidative-stress damage high blood glucose causes. Oxidative stress is a fancy way of saying you've got more destructive free radicals than antioxidant defenses. You can think of it like a war.

The imbalance causes inflammation in your tissues and in your blood, which drastically increases your risk for both heart attack and stroke. Some foods predictably increase inflammation and other foods decrease it. When you focus on eating inflammation-fighting foods, you'll not only balance your blood sugar, but also improve your brain function, reduce aches and pains, slow the aging process, and reduce your risk for heart attack, stroke, and peripheral vascular diseases.

Dieticians often guide people on how many carbohydrates they can have, and tell people to eat something every three hours. However, eating a diet of simple carbohydrate-rich meals or snacks every three hours will *never* give your body a chance to decrease your insulin level. The key factor in controlling Type 2 Diabetes is to reduce the insulin surges. So, avoiding those starchy foods and only eating three meals per day is necessary.

The diet I recommend is based on the Paleo diet. It gives you a variety of delicious foods. You'll be eating three meals a day, getting protein, vegetables, and good oils at each of those three meals. Eating this way will keep your blood sugar normal and balanced all day. It'll also keep your insulin level low enough for glucagon (the fat burning hormone) to do its job. The biggest key to the eating plan is keeping your blood sugar stable all day and all night.

The Paleo diet is a good example of this style of eating. It's an effort to eat like we used to eat back in the day...WAY back in the day. If a caveman couldn't eat it, neither can we. This means anything we could hunt or find - meats, fish, nuts, leafy greens, regional veggies, and seeds. I don't agree with everything in the Paleo diet, but many of its guidelines, especially the lean meats, good oils, and LOTS of vegetables, will really help you keep your blood sugar balanced. Eating this way once you start your detoxification will usually bring your blood glucose number down quickly. Such as Victor from chapter two. His morning blood glucose numbers came down from the 180's to the 90's in one week. This way of eating will help you regulate your glucose levels no matter how long you've had blood sugar issues. The beautiful thing about eating this way is you won't need to weigh your food or count carbohydrates either. It'll even allow your body to heal, since you will be taking in good nutrition over a long period of time. Healthy foods for the rest of your life.

Breakfast is commonly the hardest meal of the day to change. How do we make it easy, yet still healthy and within the parameters of the Paleo diet? A simple solution is a morning smoothie that includes a half a cup of fruit, a full cup of greens (spinach, kale, spring mix of greens), protein powder and either walnuts or a piece of avocado. Just add water and blend.

"I struggled with my energy levels throughout the day. Trying to find ways to stay alert after noon. I struggled to fall asleep and stay asleep and I also fluctuated with my weight.

I have only been on the program for 3 weeks, but my energy levels are consistently strong throughout the day. I only eat 3 meals a day where I use to eat 5 to 6 meals a day. Sleep is gradually getting better.

My biggest health success so far is I don't have to rely on coffee or any other pick me up stimulants for my energy levels. Since my energy levels are strong I can push myself harder during my training period and my focus is gradually improving as well! Thanks, "

Jemel J. Age 43 The Colony, TX

Healing sounds great right about now. But will I have to give up all the foods I love?

Yes and no. At the beginning, when you're at your worst, you've got to set aside any foods that are increasing your blood sugar, dragging you down, or making you worse. They may not even be foods you love, which is great. There are many other foods that *will* bring you good health. The trap for many people with food is using it to feel happy or loved. It is interesting that most 'comfort' food is *beige*.

That's right, beige potatoes, bread, bagels, rice, pasta, crackers, chips, etc. they are all variations of beige. There is no water in them and they have very little nutrient value. Yet people eat beige foods expecting to feel vibrant and energetic. To have high energy and vibrant vitality you must eat foods with naturally bright colors, and are naturally full of water, especially vegetables all the colors of a rainbow. There are better ways to feel the emotions of happiness and love. Go do something fun, go to movie, take a trip somewhere you've always wanted to go, buy yourself some flowers, spend time with friends or work in your garden. Play with a pet or try something new, such as paint, write, learn a new hobby, or meet new people. Whatever you enjoy, take some special time to do it, rather than reaching for food.

As you get healthier, your body will also be able to handle a 'treat' every once in a while. Understand that one serving of food that is not on your diet can affect your blood sugar for up to *two weeks*. So, you can't go crazy with it, but you don't have to be a zealot about your diet for the rest of your life either. We've found that strict diets don't really work anyway. People fall back into their old habits even deeper when their diets are too strict.

Remember, this is a systemized, easy to follow approach. My goal is to teach you how to become independently healthy. Others have succeeded, and you can too!

Tool of Health #3 – Hormone Balance

How do my hormones affect my blood sugar?

There are so many hormones and chemical reactions in your body - and they all have to work together. If you only did the detoxification, diet, and exercise sections, you'll probably get some good results, but you'll still plateau on weight, energy level and overall health. That's when people say things like, *"Well, how come I'm still tired?"* *"Why do I still have some weight on me?"* *"How come I'm still not sleeping well?"* or *"Why do I still feel a little bit depressed?"*

Hormones are often the hidden answer. For example, men's blood sugar issues cause their testosterone to convert to estrogen. They end up losing muscle mass and hair on their lower legs, and increasing the size of their belly. Women who have a blood sugar problem cause estrogen to convert to testosterone, and have increased hair on their chin and more menopausal symptoms. When men or women have testosterone or estrogen imbalances, they're not going to get the weight off or the shape they want, so it is vitally important to get these in balance. Testing testosterone and estrogen levels can be done via a blood test or a simple saliva test. (See the Appendix)

Hypothyroidism is another health condition needing hormone balancing. People with low thyroid function struggle to lose weight, balance their blood sugar, and have a healthy digestive tract. In fact, spikes and drops in insulin block thyroid hormones from working. Low thyroid function can also partially explain foggy thinking and difficulty losing weight - even when doing all the right diet and exercise. Remember, getting your blood glucose numbers into the good range isn't enough for optimal health, your whole body needs to become healthy.

Cortisol is another hormone that often needs balancing. You may have heard of it. It's made in the adrenal glands and is sometimes called the 'belly fat' hormone. It also regulates your sleeping and waking cycles, so if you're having trouble sleeping at night - either falling asleep, or waking up in the middle of the night and having a hard time falling asleep again - you may have a cortisol issue. Or maybe you're one of those people who just can't seem to get going in the morning. That can also be a cortisol issue. Cortisol directly affects your body's ability to recognize insulin and therefore affects your blood sugar. There is a simple saliva test you can do which measures your cortisol levels and the health of your adrenal glands. (See the Appendix)

You might be wondering how to balance your hormones or increase the health of your organs and glands. This is not something that can be done effectively with prescription medications. It is most effectively done using nutraceuticals, which are specific vitamin, mineral, herbal formulations. Because there are so many brands, so many formulations and so many possible health issues I will not give you a specific list to take here in this book. The purpose of the nutraceuticals is to increase your level of health to the point where you possibly no longer need to take them. A good licensed functional medicine health professional will look at your symptoms, lab work and what your goals are regarding your health and then make a recommendation. The bottom line is that there is no one supplement or formulation that is the 'magic pill' perfect for everyone.

Tool of Health #4 - Exercise

I feel so tired. Do I really have to exercise too?

Many people with Type 2 Diabetes are told to do some kind of cardiovascular activity. Doctors say, *"Go for a run, a bike ride, swim, or something else where your heart really kicks up its pace and you burn a lot of calories in one session."* The big caution here is that intense, prolonged exercise may bring your blood sugar down too fast, which isn't good for people with unstable blood sugar. Cardiovascular exercise early on in a recovery program will likely also cause dangerous drops in insulin. This is why exercise is the fourth tool in the system, not the first.

On top of that, many diabetics aren't even healthy enough to begin an exercise routine. If you're so fatigued that your average daily energy is only 50-60% compared to your younger days, then forcing yourself to exercise isn't in your best interest. You must get your internal organs and glands healthy first - especially your digestion and adrenal glands. At that point, you'll start feeling like you want to exercise and can then learn how exercise works as a tool to give you more blood sugar control.

As someone with Type 2 Diabetes, *muscle-building* exercises are the best for you. Building muscle doesn't take that long, and it won't cause a sudden blood sugar drop compared to cardiovascular exercise. You can do these exercises for half an hour, two to three times per week. You'll burn calories during your exercise time *and* all day long, well into the night. That means your blood sugar level will also stay more stable that whole time. And the extra muscle will burn more calories when you're not exercising, which is great if you need to lose weight.

I didn't realize adding some muscle would help so much. What's the best way to build muscle fast?

There are three great ways to build muscle. One option is going to a gym to use their weight machines. Weight machines are ideal, especially when you know how to use the equipment (many gyms have staff trained to show you how to use the equipment, just ask.) Weightlifting to build some muscle isn't 'body building.' Simply adding 5 pounds of muscle goes a long way to balancing blood sugar and getting rid of fat. That's probably a relief if you're a woman afraid you are going to end up looking like a man!

Here's a sample of a simple muscle-building routine. You can do this with any muscle group: your arms, legs, back, or abdominals.
- Set a timer for three minutes. You can use your smart phone timer, if you have one.
- Do 8 to 12 repetitions slowly, holding the contraction for two seconds when fully contracted.

- Do those 8 to 12 repetitions within the three minutes, resting for any remaining time.
- Set your timer for another three minutes, and do another 8 to 12 repetitions in the same way.
- Again, rest for the remainder of the three minutes when you're done the repetitions.
- For the final round do as many repetitions as you can, holding for two seconds when the muscle is fully contracted, until you can't do any more repetitions (your muscles 'fail'). No timer is used in this set of repetitions.

Your muscles may shake. You may feel a slight burning sensation in your muscles too. And you may feel weak after, with soreness the next day or the day after that. The good news is you'll get less and less sore as you build muscle. This type of exercise is what will give you the shape and posture you may be wanting. You'll get rid of your belly fat and be able to stand up straighter. Don't be surprised if people around you take notice and say things like, "*Wow, what are you doing? You look so great!*" How's that for a side effect?

The second option is using free weights at home. Free weights are pretty affordable, and you can get them at many different sporting goods stores. Start with 5 to 10 pounds using the same repetition sequence listed above until you're no longer sore and your body is used to doing the exercise motions. At about the 3-week mark you can start increasing the weights. To prevent injury, DO NOT start with heavy weights, with either free weights or machines.

The third option to build muscle is using gravity for resistance. It's fantastic because you can do it anywhere, hardly needing any equipment. If you travel, for example, you can use what's already in your hotel room. The best book I've seen for this was written by Mark Lauren titled *You Are Your Own Gym*. He teaches gravity-based muscle-building exercises that are excellent, fun, and challenging. These are simple exercises, such as pushups, abdominal crunches, planks, pull-ups, squats and lunges. He has a specific 10-week program that takes you through the basics. It steps you through the beginner and then the intermediate workouts to really build muscle fast.

Start off slowly to get familiar with how to do the exercises. I suggest you spend a little time looking at the pictures and reading the instructions, as I did, before getting started. These exercises are more difficult than free weights or weight machines, so go gently at first.

Tool of Health #5 – Nervous System Balance

My nervous system affects my blood sugar?

Your nervous system is a complex collection of nerves and specialized cells, called neurons, which transmit signals all over your body. Your nervous system is essentially your body's electrical wiring system. It's the master system that controls every body function, including every organ and gland. For example, your nervous system tells your pancreas how many digestive enzymes to make and when.

When your nervous system isn't balanced, your organs and glands won't receive the signals to do their jobs correctly. Your nervous system can stop working correctly for many reasons, like brain inflammation, head or spine injury, illness, or plain lack of use. As the old saying goes, "*If you don't use it, you lose it.*" This is especially true with your nervous system.

You can balance your nervous system in several ways. The first is exercise. Movement, especially balancing exercises, stimulates your nervous system. In my office, we have whole-body vibration machines (made by V-Max) that our participants stand on for 10 minutes at a time. The V-max machines cause involuntarily muscle contractions, unlike the voluntary muscle contractions from the muscle-building exercises in Tool #3. The platform you stand on oscillates in a tiny range up and down extremely fast, which engages all major muscle groups. The intense vibration also stimulates balance, coordination, core muscle strength, bone density, and detoxification.

People really like these machines since the process is quick, easy, and doesn't require changing into exercise clothes. Kirsten, who had bone density loss, purchased a V-max for her home and uses it every day. The result is that she has gone from being diagnosed with osteoporosis in her spine and both hips to having osteopenia in only one hip. She stands straighter, has more muscle and her balance and coordination are better. Visit their website www.vmaxfitness.com to find out more information about the V-max machines. If you use the promo code DRLAURA you can get a 10% discount off your order.

What's a physical chiropractic adjustment?

The second way to balance your nervous system is through chiropractic adjustments. Every adjustment is hands-on. Sometimes chiropractors use the Activator Method, so-named because it uses an instrument called an activator to make the adjustment with light tap. It uses a combination of body mechanics, neurological reflexes, and leg length tests to check your overall spinal balance and help locate your spinal misalignments. There's also a versatile hand-held device called an ArthroStim® for adjustments. Various specialized tables can help too, with various associated techniques. And then there's the classic hands-on approach to adjusting your joints. The spinal joints are generally where adjustments need to be done. Spinal adjustments are especially important to keep your muscles, organs, and glands working properly.

Why? It is important because the nerves going to every part of your body come out from the protection of your spinal column. For example, let's say the joints in your mid-back area between your shoulder blades are stuck. That's going to affect your heart and lung function. Another example is your low back. Some of the nerves there go down through your legs all the way to your toes, while some others go to your digestive tract, which can create constipation or diarrhea if not working.

You can think of your spinal joints like the little red reset buttons on electrical outlets. If you don't have them at home, think of a hotel bathroom. The electrical outlet next to the sink in the bathroom, where you plug in your electric razor or hairdryer, usually has a reset button. If you plug in your device and nothing happens, you just press the red button to reset the circuit. Chiropractic adjustments work in a similar way to reset your nervous system 'circuits' so the nerves send the proper signals, and your nervous system receives proper signals to know what's happening at all times. That way, it can respond as needed to changes. This is especially true for people like Becky, who had a lot of constipation. As long as she was adjusted on a regular basis every three to five weeks she had regular daily bowel movements. Before having chiropractic adjustments she would have a bowel movement only once every four to six days and feel very uncomfortable as a result.

The third way to balance your nervous system is taking the right supplements. There are three minerals required for every signal ever sent through any nerve: magnesium, potassium, and calcium. Your blood lab results will reveal if you have the right amounts. If you're low on any of them, you'll need to take oral supplements to boost them up.

Type 2 Diabetes and food sensitivities can cause huge inflammation all over your body, including in your brain. Inflammation in the brain is one of the causes of Alzheimer's disease. You learned with Tool #2 that I recommend a diet full of vegetables, lean meats, and 'good' oils. These oils are the anti-inflammatory oils, such as olive, flax, fish, walnut, and avocado. Eating these oils will reduce inflammation long-term and help your brain to function at its best. The fastest-working natural anti-inflammatories are ginger and curcumin (the extract of turmeric), both of which you can take in capsule form. You can also take both for as long you want. Neither will damage your liver or kidneys, unlike the over-the-counter non-steroidal anti-inflammatory drug (NSAIDS).

I see how blood sugar can affect my nervous system. Tell me why is controlling my blood sugar so important to my nervous system?

The reason is because of Type 3 Diabetes. Have you heard of Type 3 Diabetes?

Type 3 Diabetes is SCARY!!! It is Type 2 Diabetes in your brain causing Alzheimer's. It's where your brain cells no longer recognize insulin, and therefore those cells die because they can't get glucose inside to provide energy. A person with Type 2 Diabetes is 60 to 65% more likely to end up with Type 3 Diabetes. You can't bring those brain cells back to life and you can't reverse Type 3 Diabetes, but you can darn sure control your blood sugar as much as possible to prevent Type 3 Diabetes!

Can you summarize the basic steps in this system?

Sure. You have just learned the basic steps of the step-by-step system and the five main tools used to drastically increase your health and get control of your blood sugar: Detoxification, Diet, Hormone Balance, Exercise and Nervous System Balance.

This is not a process you can do once and then say you are 'cured.' These steps involve changing habits and lifestyle through continued commitment.

To keep your commitment to getting healthy, always remember your reasons for wanting to be healthy. Getting off your medications, sleeping well, having good energy, and losing weight are all wonderful and worthy of attention. It is also so important to be able to spend time with your children or grandchildren, and avoid serious health complications that cause you to become a burden to your family. The deeper level of this is living a good quality of life for the whole length of your life.

Chapter 5: How do I measure my progress?

In this chapter, we will cover which numbers to measure/test to know if you're controlling your blood sugar - and staying healthy. Keeping track of your numbers is CRITICAL. There are five specific sets of numbers to look at:

1. your daily glucose
2. Hemoglobin A1C number
3. weight
4. % body fat
5. Metabolic Assessment Questionnaire

This chapter will explain what each of these is and their relative importance. Throw out the idea of having 'good' or 'bad' numbers. This is about looking at the trends in your numbers to see your progress.

What's my morning fasting glucose number?

Your morning fasting glucose number, also called 'fasting blood glucose,' tells you how much glucose (sugar) is in your blood after not eating overnight. That's why this test is commonly used to detect diabetes, because the glucose will be high in the morning if there is no insulin or if insulin is not being recognized. The blood sample can be taken at home, at a lab, at a physician's office, or in a hospital. The normal lab range for blood glucose is 70 to 100 mg/dl. Levels between 100 and 126 mg/dl are called 'impaired fasting glucose' or 'pre-diabetes.' Diabetes is typically diagnosed when fasting blood glucose levels are 126 mg/dl or higher more than 4 mornings in a row.

Self-monitoring is important because it puts you in charge. You needn't go to a lab to have it tested. You can simply go to any drugstore, talk to the pharmacist to find out which glucose testing equipment is their best, and get the test strips for it. Insurance will often cover this equipment and test strips. Regular blood glucose monitoring gives you instant feedback on your progress is working. And you'll get even more insight if you chart your glucose numbers over time.

There are two main times of day for you to test your blood sugar levels. First thing in the morning (before eating), the number should be in the optimal range, between 85 and 99 mg/dl. (Remember, optimal is when you're in the normal range *and there are no symptoms* of health issues.) The next time is about an hour or two after you've eaten. This tells you and your medical doctor how your body is responding to food intake. When looked at together, these readings indicate if you're responding to insulin, if it's time for you to reduce or come off your medication(s), and how well you're responding to the changes you are making with your health. Your daily glucose chart is so important, I recommend you do it every day throughout your program. Once off your medications you will not need to check it as often. Like Victor said in chapter two, *"That's another good thing, you don't have to be checking your levels constantly anymore."*

What does the A1C test tell me? How often do I test it?

As you learned in chapter one, the Hemoglobin A1C test is a common blood test used to diagnose Type 1 and Type 2 Diabetes and then to gauge how well you're managing your diabetes. This test is done at a lab, a physician's office, or a hospital, and reflects your average blood sugar level for the past two to three months. Specifically, the A1C test measures what percentage of your hemoglobin - a protein in red blood cells that carries oxygen - is coated with sugar (glycated). Your daily glucose numbers tell you how you are doing in the moment, like a tiny snapshot in time, your A1C number gives you a bigger picture of how you are doing over an extended period of time. The higher the A1C level, the worse your blood sugar control and the higher your risk of diabetes complications. This test is usually done every 3 months, however, as you get healthier and healthier you will eventually only need to have it tested once or twice per year.

How do I know if my weight is really normal?

You'll know your weight is normal by tracking your weight and body fat percentage. Are you within the normal weight limit? Are you obese? Are you underweight? You can find out by looking at a 'body mass index' chart, like the one below:

Weight in Pounds

Height	100	110	120	130	140	150	160	170	180	190	200	210	220	230	240	250
4'	30.5	33.6	36.6	39.7	42.7	45.8	48.8	51.9	54.9	58.0	61.0	64.1	67.1	70.2	73.2	76.3
4'2"	28.1	30.9	33.7	36.6	39.4	42.2	45.0	47.8	50.6	53.4	56.2	59.1	61.9	64.7	67.5	70.3
4'4"	26.0	28.6	31.2	33.8	36.4	39.0	41.6	44.2	46.8	49.4	52.0	54.6	57.2	59.8	62.4	65.0
4'6"	24.1	26.5	28.9	31.3	33.8	36.2	38.6	41.0	43.4	45.8	46.2	50.6	53.0	55.4	57.9	60.3
4'8"	22.4	24.7	26.9	29.1	31.4	33.6	35.9	38.1	40.4	42.6	44.8	47.1	49.3	51.6	53.8	56.0
4'10"	20.9	23.0	25.1	27.2	29.3	31.3	33.4	35.5	37.6	39.7	41.8	43.9	46.0	48.1	50.2	52.2
5'	19.5	21.5	23.4	25.4	27.3	29.3	31.2	33.2	35.2	37.1	39.1	41.0	43.0	44.9	46.9	48.8
5'2"	18.3	20.1	21.9	23.8	25.6	27.4	29.3	31.1	32.9	34.7	36.6	38.4	40.2	42.1	43.9	45.7
5'4"	17.2	18.9	20.6	22.3	24.0	25.7	27.5	29.2	30.9	32.6	34.3	36.0	37.8	39.5	41.2	42.9
5'6"	16.1	17.8	19.4	21.0	22.6	24.2	25.8	27.4	29.0	30.7	32.3	33.9	35.5	37.1	38.7	40.3
5'8"	15.2	16.7	18.2	19.8	21.3	22.8	24.3	25.8	27.4	28.9	30.4	31.9	33.4	35.0	36.5	38.0
5'10"	14.3	15.8	17.2	18.7	20.1	21.5	23.0	24.4	25.8	27.3	28.7	30.1	31.6	33.0	34.4	35.9
6'	13.6	14.9	16.3	17.6	19.0	20.3	21.7	23.1	24.4	25.8	27.1	28.5	29.8	31.2	32.5	33.9
6'2"	12.8	14.1	15.4	16.7	18.0	19.3	20.5	21.8	23.1	24.4	25.7	27.0	28.2	29.5	30.8	32.1
6'4"	12.2	13.4	14.6	15.8	17.0	18.3	19.5	20.7	21.9	23.1	24.3	25.6	26.8	28.0	29.2	30.4
6'6"	11.6	12.7	13.9	15.0	16.2	17.3	18.5	19.6	20.8	22.0	23.1	24.3	25.4	26.6	27.7	28.9
6'8"	11.0	12.1	13.2	14.3	15.4	16.5	17.6	18.7	19.8	20.9	22.0	23.1	24.2	25.3	26.4	27.5
6'10"	10.5	11.5	12.5	13.6	14.6	15.7	16.7	17.8	18.8	19.9	20.9	22.0	23.0	24.0	25.1	26.1
7'	10.0	11.0	12.0	13.0	13.9	14.9	15.9	16.9	17.9	18.9	19.9	20.9	21.9	22.9	23.9	24.9

Height in Feet and Inches

http://www.freebmicalculator.net

Underweight   Nomal   Overweight   Obesity

You might be surprised that Type 2 diabetics can struggle with being either overweight *or* underweight. So you might need to lose some weight, or you might need to gain some weight. And you can do both - while balancing your blood sugar - by building some lean muscle mass. The media rarely mentions skinny and normal weight people getting Type 2 Diabetes. There isn't much written about them in the scientific literature either even though it affects over 10% of Type 2 diabetics.

According to the American Diabetic Association, **one in three Type 2 diabetics aren't even diagnosed**! It's possible that many of these people are lean, so they don't even suspect they have Type 2 Diabetes. The "only fat people get diabetes" myth is one of the most dangerous of all health myths.

At some point in your program, you'll find that your weight plateaus, which can feel frustrating. That's the time to stop looking at just your weight. Instead, start looking at your body fat percentage. This number is much more important than weight, and there isn't nearly as much emotional baggage about it either.

The American Council on Exercise uses the following categories based on body fat percentage:

	Women	Men
Essential fat	10-12%	2-4%
Athletes	14-20%	6-13%
Fitness	21-24%	14-17%
Acceptable	25-31%	18-25%
Obese	32% or more	26% or more

There are many options online to determine your body fat percentage.

Most body fat calculators use the U.S. Navy's Percentage Body Fat Formula. As with all body fat calculators, it's only an estimate, but it can give fairly accurate estimates for both men and women. Here are the measurements you'll need to plug into the calculator:

Waist (Male) - Circumference around belly-button level
Waist (Female) - Circumference where you're skinniest, widthwise
Neck - Circumference of neck, with tape sloping slightly downward to the front.
Hips - Circumference where you're widest

Tracking your body fat percentage will help keep you motivated to keep building muscle, so you look and feel great without worrying about your weight.

Isn't there more to it than just numbers? How do I track my symptoms to know if I'm really getting somewhere?

Reflecting on how you feel as you go is just as important as the physical measurements. For example, if you do my program, you start by filling out a comprehensive Health Assessment Questionnaire. The questionnaire is easy to fill out and helps clarify which of your organs and glands are suffering versus which ones are doing well. You just rate how often you experience specific symptoms from 0 to 3 (0 = never, 1 = occasionally, 2 = often, 3 = all the time). You answer these questions every three months to monitor your own progress and zoom in on where you need to focus on increasing your health.

Lastly, if you've had a problem with diabetes before, diabetes can creep back up on you if you go back to your previous lifestyle habits. That's why it's important to keep checking your numbers, even after you've reversed Type 2 Diabetes. You just won't need to check them as often. You can check your glucose once a week and your A1C and body fat percentage only every six months to a year. You can also fill out the Health Assessment Questionnaire just once each year. By knowing your numbers, you'll learn how to be independently healthy without ever needing diabetes medication.

Chapter 6: When Can I Go Off The Medications?

There are so many questions about medications that this chapter is dedicated to answering the most common questions related to diabetes medications, such as, how and when to you can stop taking your medications.

"I have to confess that when my wife Ellen first dragged me to one of Dr Laura's seminars I was to say the least; skeptical. Dr. Laura's presentation was polished and informative but did little to change my mind or dispel my skepticism. However, my Ellen's blood sugar numbers had been steadily creeping up for ten years and her regular doctor's only response was to continue increasing the dosage of her diabetic medications.

One definition of insanity is to keep doing the same thing expecting different results. Additionally Ellen, generally the smarter of the two of us, saw the possibility and wanted to try Dr. Laura's program. So I tucked my skepticism away in the back of my mind, told her I would support her, and we signed up for the program.

As they say, seeing is believing and we have seen the results. Ellen has lost weight, her morning blood test numbers have fallen significantly, and for the first time in years her A1C number has actually dropped, going from 7.3 to 6.0.

Ellen's doctor has reduced the dosage on two of her medications and there is reason to believe she may be able to eliminate the diabetes medication entirely. But best of all, Ellen is healthier, feeling better, and enjoying life more.

I am no longer a skeptic. Instead I am an enthusiastic supporter and have recommended Dr Laura's program to several other people."

John & Ellen   Age 70   The Colony, TX

When can I ditch my medications?

The best way to know is by looking in your journal where you've been recording your glucose numbers, as discussed in the last chapter. In my experience, when your blood glucose is below 85 mg/dl, it's time to talk to your medical doctor about reducing your medications. That said, many people can actually start reducing their medications once their fasting glucose drops below 100 mg/dl. Keep in mind, your normal blood sugar levels should be consistently between 85 and 99 mg/dl. That's optimal.

NOTE: You must speak to your medical doctor about your medications. Their job is helping you manage your medications. My job is teaching you how to be healthy so you don't need medications.

In the ideal world, I'd never take another drug. But is it really safe for me to cut down on them?

Nearly everybody wonders about this. It's only natural, especially if you've been dependent on your meds. There are two reasons it's safe. First, if you've been taking medication for a while, you already know how your body responds. You know when things don't feel right in your body, and you know when you feel great.

The second reason is your regular medical doctor, who prescribed your medications, will monitor you as you reduce your dosages. Your pharmacist is also trained to answer questions about your medications. Thousands of people free themselves of medications every year. Some, like Victor, drastically reduce their dosages within days, some, like Jireh, within a few weeks, and others, like Kent, within a few months.

So should I keep taking my meds until I get my doctor's clearance not to?

Yes! Keep taking your medications until you get clearance not to from your medical doctor. As I mentioned before, medication isn't my scope of practice. That's not what I'm trained in. I'm trained to teach you how to get healthy and stay healthy. I *highly* recommend you tell your medical doctor in advance that you are starting a program to alert them that you will need their help. When you go in to see them, show them your glucose readings chart and the other numbers you've been recording, so you can get advice on which medication to go off of first and by how much. You may also get a pat on the back for doing a great job.

What would happen if I stopped taking my medications now?

DON'T quit your medications before starting this program because your body will be unprepared for the sudden changes. You might end up in the emergency room in a coma from sky-high blood sugar. Take things step by step instead. Tell your medical doctor before you start any program. Once you've started detoxifying, eating how I teach in my program, and your glucose numbers are in the optimal 85 to 99 mg/dl range, or even below 85 mg/dl, you can talk to your medical doctor about reducing your medications. That's because you know your body is healing, when your glucose numbers are in range. And that only happens when your body is recognizing insulin again.

What about my non-diabetes meds? When can I stop taking those?

Only your prescribing medical doctor can answer that definitively. I'll give you the same answer whether you're talking about your diabetes medications (Metformin, Lantis, Actose, Januvia, Glipizide, Janumet, Humalog etc.) or your cholesterol, blood pressure, thyroid, or other medications. Each of these has different associated numbers to monitor and often different sets of symptoms. When your symptoms and lab work start improving ask to speak with your doctor to reduce or go off of certain medications.

Reducing any kind of medication depends on the kinds of medications you're taking and why you're taking them in the first place. Many people come off of some or all of their diabetes medications within two to eight weeks of starting my 12 week program. In contrast, it usually takes several months to heal enough to come off of cholesterol, blood pressure, (like Mike did in chapter three) and antidepressant medications.

Again, NEVER self-prescribe your medication dosages. Talk with your medical doctor before you make any changes.

Are there herbs I can take instead of medications?

Some studies indicate the herbs such as berberine or cinnamon can take the place of metformin. The problem with doing this is that you are replacing one drug for another and long-term neither will actually help you to increase your health.

Other herbs such as Gymnema sylvestre, Bitter Melon Extract, and Banaba Extract can be very helpful in actually helping your body to heal. Ask your licensed natural health provider about these for further information.

Chapter 7: What Makes This Permanent?

Will my health always be good?

Your health will be good because you're going to shift your habits. Type 2 Diabetes isn't a genetic issue, as many people believe. It just *looks* like it's genetic because who do we learn our diet and exercise habits from? That's right: we learn them from our family, our parents, grandparents, and so on. Sometimes the habits are deeply ingrained in our culture. For example, there are many different cultures with much higher rates of Type 2 Diabetes than other cultures. The more your main cultural staples are based on simple carbohydrates, like bread, rice, potatoes, pasta, tortillas, and very sweet desserts, the higher your risk.

Here's an analogy to help you understand how this program can make a permanent difference in your life. For example, if you want increase your ability to speak a foreign language you might take a class to learn that language better. The more you practice by speaking the new language the more fluent you become. If you don't use the new words and phrases over and over that you learned you will eventually forget them.

That's what this program is like. You are learning the language, of how to increase your health. To maintain that health you must continue to use the new habits that you learned, or you will slide backward with your health. The most important concept in this book is consistency with your new habits. These are lifestyle changes for the rest of your life.

That's how the changes become permanent. When you learn new habits such as the five Health Tools mentioned in chapter four (detoxification, diet, exercise, and making sure your hormones and your nervous system are balanced), your old ways of thinking and doing things fade away. The ultimate goal is to teach you how to have freedom and become independent with your health for life, including from medications. Sure, it's still important to consult with a doctor on occasion, too, but that's for routine checkups.

That sounds great, Doc. But will the lifestyle changes be *forever*? That still sounds too hard.

Many people ask variants of your question... *"Do I always have to eat this way?" "What if I miss a week of exercise?" "What if I'm going on vacation or it's my birthday or special holiday?" "Can I have a treat every now and then?" "Can I have a glass of wine with dinner?" "Can I have a piece of cake at an office party?"* All good questions. Here's another analogy: If you have a fire in your fireplace and all you do is add wood, add wood, and add more wood, and you never clean out the ashes, pretty soon you'll have a fireplace full of ashes. There won't even be room to have a fire. It's going to be an inefficient mess. Eventually, the ashes will start falling out of the fireplace and smudge your rugs, furniture, walls and house pets (yikes!). This is what happens in your body when glucose and toxins build up your metabolic pathways. Everything stop working right.

So, what you've got to do, especially at the beginning, is stop the fire and clean out the ashes. Then, after several months of sticking with your healthy habits, every once in a while, if you want to have a fire in fireplace, have a fire! Enjoy a glass of wine. Eat a piece of bread. You'll know by how you feel after you've eaten those foods, as to whether you can have more or not. You'll know from your glucose levels and your A1C test results if you are doing a good job of sticking with the program.

If you do "fall of the wagon - or underneath it" you now know how to clean out the ashes and get right back on course. You'll also be certain that the habit changes you've made have permanently changed your body, so you won't have to take medication or rely on any specific doctor for your health.

Let me be clear, you will *never* be able to go back to eating sugar and simple carbohydrates daily, that's part of what caused the problem to begin with. However, you will be able to have some on occasion. When people feel healthy energetic and happy they don't want to go back to the way they were. You will be living a healthy, energetic, happy, and purposeful life by following this program. No more living in fear, you'll be living in freedom.

Feeling good and having energy would be a dream come true. So how will I *know* if the positive changes are permanent?

You'll know your changes are permanent by looking at your lab numbers for glucose, A1C, and percent body fat, plus periodically filling out the health assessment questionnaire. Seeing how consistently balanced these results are will tell you how lasting the changes are. You'll compare your daily glucose numbers and your A1C numbers, to previous tests. You'll know your changes have become permanent when your numbers are consistently in range. Eventually, you can check A1C only once a year, as long as you stick with the improved lifestyle habits.

How you know that you have learned something from this program is how your health habits will be different from this point on. *If you don't change any habits, you didn't learn anything.*

If you keep doing the same thing you've always done, you're going to keep getting the same results you've always gotten. For things to change, you have to change. Things get better by purposeful change, they don't get better by chance.

One of our biggest enemies is sliding backward into our old habits. Here are important questions to ask yourself to help you continue to reach your goals, and NOT slide backwards into old habits.

1. How has your health and your life changed as a result of implementing this program?
2. How have you EXPERIENCED the difference?
3. How do you feel when you stray from this program?

Experiencing the difference in your health and being consistent with your new habits is the most important part of this program.

Chapter 8: Time To Take Action

Hope For Reversing Your Diabetes

Diabetes is a debilitating disease because of the countless complications it can cause when not properly managed. Diabetes can cause issues with your circulation, eyes, gum health, kidneys, and heart, to name a few. Severe complications can lead to heart attacks, strokes, blindness, amputation of your legs or arms, and it can lead to death from kidney failure. It can be hard to know where to start in increasing your health and, unfortunately, traditional medicine is trained to treat diabetes with medications. Some participants express that they feel trapped with their health, because these medications often leave them feeling worse and no one ever told them there was a way out.

Type 1 Diabetics have to inject insulin for the rest of their lives because their bodies don't make insulin anymore. As a Type 2 diabetic you have power over your situation, and you must be proactive about your blood sugar levels to avoid becoming dependent on insulin shots - as in Double Diabetes. That said, people with Type 2 Diabetes *can* control their blood sugar and with the proper eating and lifestyle habits, like Dean, Victor, Jireh, Mike, and Lisa who were all mentioned in this book, as well as thousands of others.

I know I need to take action, where do I begin?

There are two quick, simple and easy ways to take action right now that will make a big impact.

1. Watch the free video series on my website. **www.bloodsugarideas.com**
2. Follow the system in chapter four of this book.

How is this program is different from everything else out there?

No other program covers the specific actions you can control that affect blood sugar as well as the five Health Tools that improve your whole wellbeing. Most other programs only focus on diet or taking supplements in place of medications.

1. This program helps you discover some of the root causes of why you have blood sugar issues AND guides you on what to do to take control of those causes.
2. Through this program you are taught how to track your progress in ALL the aspects of your health, not just tracking your blood sugar.
3. You have access to the information online, making it easy and convenient to fit into your lifestyle.
4. If you need help with accountability you can have an accountability call by phone each week with one of our 'Accountability Partners' so you can ask questions and get reassurance when you need it.
5. This program is more than just a book, it is an online curriculum that teaches you how to increase your health!

What will we discover in this 12 week online program?

All the information is put into an easy to follow step-by-step system that you follow each week at a time. The following is a checklist of all the things you will learn and some of the accomplishments other participants have achieved:

- ✓ Understand your blood sugar and what your lab test results mean, as well as what to do about them if they go out of range.
- ✓ Understand the devastating complications of Diabetes.
- ✓ Stop insulin surges to get control of your blood sugar without pills or shots.
- ✓ Diet where most people lose 20-50 pounds of fat so you can fit into that smaller dress size or pant size that's been hanging in your closet for years. What an incredible feeling that is!
- ✓ Learn healthy habits, so you can keep the weight off and not gain it back!
- ✓ Exercise that burns fat even while you sleep, so you look good even to yourself when you look in the mirror.
- ✓ Get a good night's sleep and wake up feeling rested.
- ✓ Increase your energy by 50 - 80%, so you feel alive again to enjoy life! Such as enjoy playing with your grandchildren without being so exhausted.
- ✓ Perform better at work and in the bedroom, so your spouse raves about you and how they have their spouse back.
- ✓ How to protect your kidneys, so that you lower your risk for kidney failure, and never have to succumb to the dialysis machine.
- ✓ Eat the foods that will also lower cholesterol and triglycerides, so you can reduce your risk for heart attack and stroke - no hospital stays or expenses.
- ✓ Identify food sensitivities and remove the foods that cause inflammation from your diet
- ✓ Discover how digestion can cause blood sugar spikes, and by correcting this one thing you can also get rid of acid reflux and decrease your risk for esophagus cancer.
- ✓ Reduce having to prick yourself to check your blood sugar several times in a day, no more pain, buying expensive lancets or test strips - you may never have to prick yourself again.
- ✓ Never have to worry about amputation or being stuck in a wheelchair, so you will always have your ability to walk on

your own two feet, and have independence for the rest of your life.

✓ Have improved vision, decrease your risk of blindness, and be able to watch your grandchildren grow - drive them around and NOT have your car and driver's license taken away from you.

✓ Exercise the quickest easiest way, while keeping your blood sugar stable.

✓ Cut your list of medications and stop insulin shots in their tracks.

✓ Feel like your normal self again, and be able to enjoy being with your friends, family, and where you volunteer.

✓ Reduce your risk of Type 3 Diabetes, keep your mental faculties strong.

✓ Gain self confidence, self respect, the respect of your peers.

✓ Have independence with your health for the rest of your life.

How do we achieve those great results using this program?

The best results are achieved by following the system step-by-step, each week at a time, each new habit at a time. Watching the videos and having an 'Accountability Partner' really make a big difference in achieving results.

"I thought that my health was in good shape; however, it was really somewhere between fair and poor before I started the program.

I have been on the program one and half months (1.5) and my health is improving daily. My health is now in the GOOD range and gets better daily. I have been able to stop over half of my prescription medicine and am eating much healthier foods/diet than I have in my life.

My biggest health success so far: I found a program that understands my body and its challenges. This has allowed me to begin the changes for a healthier life style and renewed health.

Thank you for teaching me how to get my life back and to live longer!"

Tito K   Age 60   Allen, TX

Who is this program best suited for?

The 12 week "Diabetes Turning Point Program" that this book is based on is perfect for you if you(r):

- Have been told you're Pre-Diabetic or Type 2 Diabetic.
- Have been told to watch your diet and do some exercise.
- Not sure what to do to lose weight or what kind of diet or exercise is best for you.
- Need to lose 20-50 lbs.
- Are grumpy or cranky or tired a lot.
- Have tried other plans and you are not sure what to do next.
- Are concerned about the scary complications of Type 2 Diabetes: heart attack, stroke, kidney failure, blindness, amputation, or diabetic neuropathy, Type 3 Diabetes.
- Already have open sores on your feet or legs that won't heal or you've had toes amputated.
- Not sleeping well - can't fall asleep, wake up and can't go back to sleep, or getting up multiple times the night to pee.
- Don't want to end up like your aging parents with their health issues.
- Are taking diabetes medications or shots.
- Tired of making sure that you have your meds and when you have to get refills.
- Are feeling isolated and unmotivated to do the things you used to enjoy.
- Want to enjoy playing with your grandchildren without being so exhausted.
- Notice a loss of quality of life and zest for life, mildly depressed.
- Want to feel like your normal self again.
- Want to maintain a certain level of quality health for as long as possible and you know that to achieve that level of

health you must get better control of your blood sugar.

If, you resonate with any of these fears or needs, I suggest you start this program immediately!

This program is *not* for you if you(r):

- Don't have a blood sugar issue.
- Are not willing to take responsibility for your health.
- Are unwilling to change your habits.
- Don't need to lose weight, are sleeping well, and have lots of energy.
- Believe that medication will cure you.
- Doctor says you are in perfect health and you don't need any medications of any kind.

You have asked me a lot of great questions throughout this book, and now I, Dr. Shwaluk, want to ask you a question.

Are you ready to take action?

You have a choice to make regarding your health. We've talked about the destructive complications of diabetes and I'm asking you clearly how do you want to end up in life?

Do you want to end up: overmedicated with pills and shots, can't move because you are too fat and winded, are riddled with pain and stiffness, can't feel your feet, no libido, run the risks of stroke, amputation, heart attack, being hooked up to a dialysis machine, can't get around because you are in a wheelchair, can't see anyone because you are blind, can't drive or be independent, all your money goes to pay medical bills, stuck in a bed in a long term care facility, and you feel depressed.

Do you want that? Or would you rather...

Learn how to eat the right foods, do the right exercise, have weight come off and keep it off, control your blood sugar, decrease medication, reduce your risk of any serious health issues (heart attack, stroke, blindness, amputation, kidney failure) and have energy for your whole life, living to a fulfilled ripe old age with all your faculties, so you can fulfill your purpose in life and say "I love you" one more time to the people you care about?

The choice is yours. It's up to you to take the next easy steps.

1. Watch the free video series on my website. **www.bloodsugarideas.com**
2. Follow the system in chapter four of this book.

7 Secrets to Having Your BEST Health EVER!!!

When People Focus On What It Takes To Be Healthy They Gain Health For Life With These Seven Simple Steps

1. Understand where you are at with your health. This means learning what the optimal ranges are for your lab work, rather than the disease ranges.

2. Free yourself of *thinking* that medications are going to increase your health when it comes to most chronic diseases. You are the one who needs to put in the effort.

3. Focus on building up your knowledge on the 5 Tools of Health – Detoxification, Nutrition, Exercise, Hormone and Nervous System Function.

4. Plan for success. Plan your day, week, month in advance so that you are prepared to succeed at being healthy.

5. IMPLEMENT what you learn into your daily habits.

6. Be consistent! Choose the same good habits EVERY day, not just some days.

7. Keep in mind that being healthy is not a short journey, it is a journey for LIFE!

Letter From The Author

I've worked in the alternative healthcare industry one-on-one with people since 1996. I have a bachelors of science in cellular, molecular and microbial biology from the University of Calgary in Alberta Canada, a Doctorate in Chiropractic, and post graduate education in Applied Kinesiology, Functional Nutrition And Functional Endocrinology. I am licensed with the Pastoral Medical Association. I've authored 2 books, have done multiple TV and radio interviews, and have done 1000's of live classes and speaking engagements over the last 20 years.

I'd like to share with you how this life saving program began...

It all started with a few people one-on-one in my office who wanted get healthy to see if they could get off their diabetes medications. They didn't want to have to stick themselves with needles for insulin or take any medications at all, and what I suggested for them really worked out well. Soon I was teaching 15 to 20 people a month every month with this program. Then someone said, "*This program has really taught me a lot Dr. Shwaluk and I wish you would put it online so that my brother and sister, who live at opposite ends of the country, can get the success with their health that I got.*"

I said, "*Okay*" and I started writing and making videos. During lunch hour every day I wrote and I wrote, and on weekends and after work I made videos to demonstrate everything and how to do everything. My husband even helped me by doing more stuff at home so that I could create the program and get it done with good quality information.

When I mentioned the "Diabetes Turning Point Program" to people they wanted in before I even got it finished! When I did finish putting everything together in the online format I thought it was good. It worked for many people who went through the program for the very first time with HUGE successes. We made some updates to make it even better, more user friendly and informative. Then I started selling it online. I'm very excited to present it to you now at **www.bloodsugarideas.com**

I can't tell you the amount of pleasure I felt when I received my first success letter from Jerry L. in Texas.

> *"Thank each and everyone there,*
> *for great support, and tools to*
> *LIVE LIFE ONCE AGAIN!!!!"*

Soon we were getting emails from England, Canada and Germany asking for this program. Since then, I've gotten hundreds more of those letters.

I welcome your success letter too. Please send it to me via email at support@bloodsugarideas.com or in the mail to 2540 East Plano Pkwy #142, Plano TX 75074, USA

Your doctor for health,
Dr. Laura Shwaluk

Appendix of Lab Tests

Cyrex Labs Array 10 Multiple Food Immune Reactivity Screen

Food sensitivities can not only cause a lot of gut issues, they can increase your blood sugar numbers! Many of our participants test for food sensitivities to find out which foods are affecting the state of their health! This is a very simple blood test that checks over 200 different kinds of foods.

The Adrenal Stress Index (ASI)

This panel was introduced in 1989 to evaluate stress, a leading cause of morbidity and mortality. Additional tests have been added to evaluate glycemic control using multiple salivary insulin measurements, and to evaluate adrenal capacity to produce cortisol using 17-Hydroxyprogesterone. The Diagnos-Techs™ Adrenal Stress Index (ASI) is a non-invasive way to help evaluate the effects of stress on your body. It includes 10 tests for six different hormones and immune markers that may be affected by chronic stress or other conditions.

The Adrenal Stress Index can:
• Help to identify possible causes of excessive fatigue
• Help your physician understand how to reduce your food cravings and build and maintain muscle mass
• Identify underlying reasons for chronic infections such as sinusitis or other recurrent respiratory infections
• Help your doctor to determine if a gluten-free diet may be right for you
• Identify possible reasons why you may have difficulty falling asleep or staying asleep

Four saliva samples are used to assess the following:
-Cortisol Helps evaluate the stress response
-Insulin Helps investigate blood sugar control
-DHEA/DHEA-S Helps determine degree to which other hormones may be affected by cortisol changes
-Secretory IgA Helps evaluate the toll of stress on immunity
-17-OH progesterone Helps determine underlying causes of abnormal cortisol levels
-Gluten antibodies Helps identify immune response to gluten

Comprehensive Metabolic Panel
This is the comprehensive blood test that I recommend.

Labcorp reference number 346029   Opti-K-Plex 2 Panel
 (Fasting / Avoid Exercise)
 Components:
 (CMP 14); Lipid Panel with LDL/HDL Ratio; Iron, Serum with Total
Iron Binding Capacity (TIBC), Percent Iron Saturation, Unsaturated Iron
Binding Capacity (UIBC); Ferritin; LDH; GGT; Magnesium, Serum;
Phosphorus, Serum; Uric Acid, Serum; Thyroid Panel with TSH;
Triiodothyronine (Total T3), Total T4; Hemoglobin A1c; C-Reactive
Protein (CRP), High Sensitivity; Vitamin D, 25-Hydroxycalciferol;
Homocysteine; Fibrinogen Activity; Complete Blood Count (CBC) with
Differential and Platelet Count; Urinalysis, Routine

Gastrointestinal Health Panel™
The GI Health Panel™ is a non-invasive screen of the gastrointestinal
tract and its function. It includes 15-22 individual, yet related tests. Stool
and saliva samples are submitted by the patient after home collection.

These tests utilize proven biochemical and state-of-the-art
immunological testing and other methods. The panel includes:

- Pathogen screening for bacteria, fungi, yeast and various
  parasites.
- Digestion-related screens for enzyme levels and
  immunochemical markers for intolerance to common
  offending foods.
- Intestinal function markers to evaluate irritation and
  inflammation; markers indicate overall status of gut
  immunity and integrity, such as occult blood.

Index

Available Programs At
www.BloodSugarIdeas.com

1. "Reverse Type 2 Diabetes FREE 5 Part Video Series!" You Will Discover…

- 3 BIG Myths about Type 2 Diabetes
- 4 Keys to Defeating Type 2 Diabetes…
- 5 Tools Used to Drastically Improve Your Health
- Drugs: The BIG Lie That's Giving You False Hope…
- Why Taking Diabetes Drugs Can (and Usually Does) Continue to Make Your Health Worse…
- According to the Centers for Disease and Drug Control: Type 2 Diabetes is Preventable and Controllable…
- Silent Killer: Why Your Lab Tests Could Be Normal, But You Still Have Pre-Diabetes or Diabetes…
- And MUCH More!

If You Have Diabetes (or Have Been Told You're Pre-Diabetic) this free video series is a MUST!

2. "Diabetes QUICK START Program" includes...

- Quick Start Guide Download
- Survey to help you get clear on your goals
- Get started videos and action items that teach you which steps you can take to increase your health and immediately start bringing your blood sugar levels back to balance
- Metabolic Assessment form to help you get to the root causes of your health issues
- One-on-one consultation with one of our health professionals to help you achieve optimal health

Everything you need to get a jump start on balancing your blood sugar FAST!

3. The 12 Week "Diabetes Turning Point Program" Includes:

- 12 weeks of online learning that opens up week by week to guide you in an easy to follow, step-by-step format
- Downloadable workbook
- Simple, quick and easy recipes and shopping guide to make your meal planning easy
- Short videos that demonstrate exactly how and what to do to balance your blood sugar without taking up too much of your time
- Information on all 14 factors that affect your blood sugar
- Charts for understanding your blood lab test results AND what to do about it if something is out of range
- Graphs that easily explain the material you are learning.
- Encouragement videos to keep you motivated
- Access to ask our health professionals questions about your program
- 12 phone calls with one of our 'Accountability Partners' who are trained to guide you step by step

Everything you need to really understand your blood sugar and how to increase your health so that you can have freedom and independence with your health for the rest of your life.

Printed in Great Britain
by Amazon